Healing Prayer Services
for Those Who Mourn

Praying Through Grief

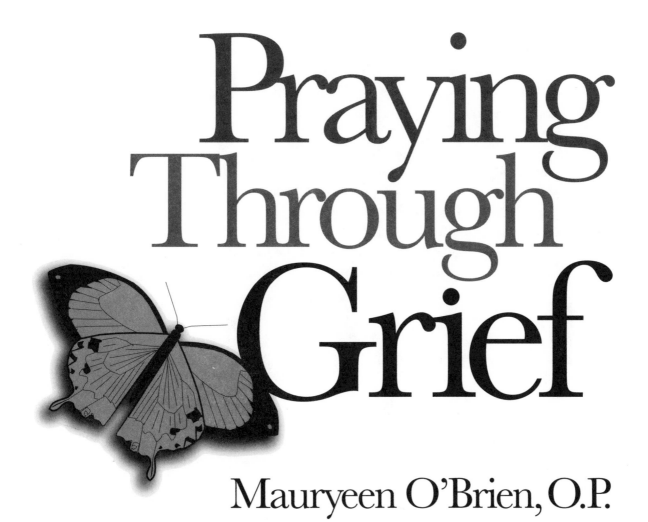

Mauryeen O'Brien, O.P.

AVE MARIA PRESS Notre Dame, Indiana 46556

Scripture quotations are from New Revised Standard Version of the Bible. Copyright © 1989 by the Division of Christian Education of the National Council of the Churches of Christ in the U.S.A. Used by permission. All rights reserved.

"The Road Not Taken" from *The Poetry of Robert Frost*, ed. by Edward Connery Lathem. Published by Henry Holt & Co., Inc. Used by permission.

"We Remember Them" from *The Gates of Prayer* by Central Conference of American Rabbis, 1975, p. 552. Used by permission.

"The Sycamore Retreat" and "Passings" from *Mortal on the Mend* by Vincent Marquis, Wallingford, CT (unpublished). Used by permisison.

"Light a Candle," music and words by Paul Alexander, Paul Alexander Music, P.O. Box 125, Rockville Centre, New York 11571, 1993. Used by permission.

"We Remember" by Marty Haugen, G.I.A. Publications, Inc., 7404 S. Mason Ave., Chicago, Illinois 60638. Reprinted by permission of G.I.A. Publications.

Excerpts from *Praying Our Goodbyes*, by Joyce Rupp, copyright 1988 by Ave Maria Press, Notre Dame, Indiana 46556, are used with permission of the publisher.

Gift From the Sea, by Anne Morrow Lindbergh © 1955, 1975 by Anne Morrow Lindbergh. Reprinted by permission of Pantheon Books, a division of Random House, Inc.

Sincere thanks to Cecelia O'Brien and Kathleen Ryzewski who prepared the manuscript for the computer.

© 1997 by Ave Maria Press, Inc.

International Standard Book Number: 0-87793-629-3

Book design by Elizabeth French

Printed and bound in the United States of America.

Library of Congress Cataloging-in-Publication Data

O'Brien, Mauryeen.
      Praying through grief : healing prayer services for those who mourn / Mauryeen O'Brien.
          p.   cm.
      Includes bibliographical references.
      ISBN 0-87793-629-3
      1. Church work with the bereaved—Catholic Church. 2. Prayer groups—Catholic Church.
   3. Catholic Church—Prayer-books and devotions—English.   I. Title.
BX2347.8.B470271997
264'.0274—dc21   97-17053
                                                          CIP

This book is dedicated to
Pat, Peggy, and Regina,
three "valiant women" who
permitted me to walk with them
on their journey to eternal life.
May they rest in peace.

Contents

Introduction

After the loss of a loved one, we can expect that we will go through some kind of a grief process. The one whom we held so dear is no longer with us, and we need to mourn that loss if we are ever to move on with our lives. That mourning will have no time limit. It will not proceed logically or step-by-step, and may hit us over and over again.

We know we have to go through our grief; there is no way around it or over it or under it. We must work through it, and that will be the hardest work we will ever attempt. Support groups and therapists and grief literature may help in getting us to face our grief. We should take advantage of them.

Prayer and ritual will also be an important part of our healing process in our journey through grief. Prayer and ritual are a central part of our existence; they provide a framework for us where through the use of repetition, familiarity, and transformation of what is known, new behaviors, actions, and meanings can occur. They mark the major moments as we move through life, and they help us to express the deepest thoughts and feelings about life's most important events. If we commemorate and celebrate birth and marriage, parenthood and ordination, why not do the same as we face the death of our loved ones, gathering together the memories that made them so very special to us?

In times of grief, prayer and ritual can bring a sense of balance and peace. They give us an opportunity to say goodbye, to express our pain, to adjust to a transition, to remember our loved ones, and to place those "remembrances" in the context of the present. They connect us with our past, define our present life, and show us a path to the future. Hopefully, they can raise our awareness so that, together with the others assembled in remembrance, a sense of transformation can take place.

No matter what we have experienced, if we are open and responsive to the depth of that experience and the mystery of it, we will begin to understand more fully the paradoxes in our lives. Life is not just happy, or just sad; life is a combination of the two. This realization can open us to the fullness of celebration. We see this over and over again in the life of Christ. The apostles certainly did not rejoice over his crucifixion and death; nor did Christ welcome it with open arms. But from that suffering and death came the opportunity to celebrate—just three days later—his *new* life, both for himself and for his apostles, and ultimately for us. And that is the essence of celebration: out of the sadness and pain of loss and unhappiness can come the joy and hope of new life. If we can celebrate that, then the new is not frightening; it is life-giving.

The celebration doesn't have to be extraordinary. It can be quiet and reflective; it can be spirited and lively. It can be anything that expresses the realization that new life is possible.

No matter how dark and frightening the nights of struggle have been after the death of our loved one, we can be assured that daylight will always come. May the prayer and ritual celebrated in this volume help us to obtain a sense of solace and healing as we set aside time to try to touch the sacred.

Notes on Using This Book

The prayer services and rituals in this book are not taken from an approved liturgical book. They are offered in the spirit of the *Constitution on the Liturgy*, no. 13, which suggests that non-liturgical devotions "harmonize with the liturgical seasons, accord with the sacred liturgy, are in some fashion derived from it, and lead the people to it."

The prayer services may be used on a variety of occasions. All may be used to commemorate the anniversary of death. For each service, particularly appropriate times for usage are noted.

These prayer services are also designed to be used in any number of different settings: in parishes, in support groups for the bereaved, in retreat settings, by families, or by individuals.

Materials needed are listed at the beginning of each prayer service. Music other than the songs listed may be substituted.

Each service is followed by a participant sheet that may be duplicated for use with this prayer service. These participant sheets may not be copied by anyone else, or for any other purpose, without the written permission of the publisher.

Resources Needed

Many of the prayer services in this book use the hymnal *Glory and Praise*. Some also call for a cassette recording of *Glory and Praise*. If you do not have these materials, check your parish resource center. Or, you may purchase them from: OCP Publications, 5536 N.E. Hassalo, Portland, OR 97213, 1-800-548-8749.

The following music publications are also mentioned in various liturgies. Any of these, however, may be replaced with any recording of meditative music.

"Ave Maria," (several versions are available on *Ave Maria*, Ave Maria Press, Notre Dame, IN 46556, 1-800-282-2865). Any rendition may be used.

"The Holly and the Ivy" (available in many collections of Christmas carols).

"Light a Candle," Paul Alexander. Tape may be purchased from Paul Alexander Music, P.O Box 125, Rockville Centre, NY 11571.

"The Lilies of the Field," by John Michael Talbot, from *Troubadour of the Great King* produced by Birdwing Music/Cherry Lane Publishing Co., Inc., Sparrow Records, Inc.

"The Path of Life," David Haas, from *Who Calls You By Name*, G.I.A. Publications, Inc., 7404 S. Mason Ave., Chicago, IL 60638, 1-708-496-3800.

"We Remember," Marty Haugen, from *With Open Hands* collection, © 1983, G.I.A. Publications, Inc., 7404 S. Mason Ave., Chicago, IL 60638, 1-708-496-3800.

"Wood Hath Hope," John Foley, S.J., from *Wood Hath Hope*, B.M.I. Recordings. Available from: OCP Publications, 5536 N.E. Hassalo, Portland, OR 97213, 1-800-548-8749.

Spring
and
Summer

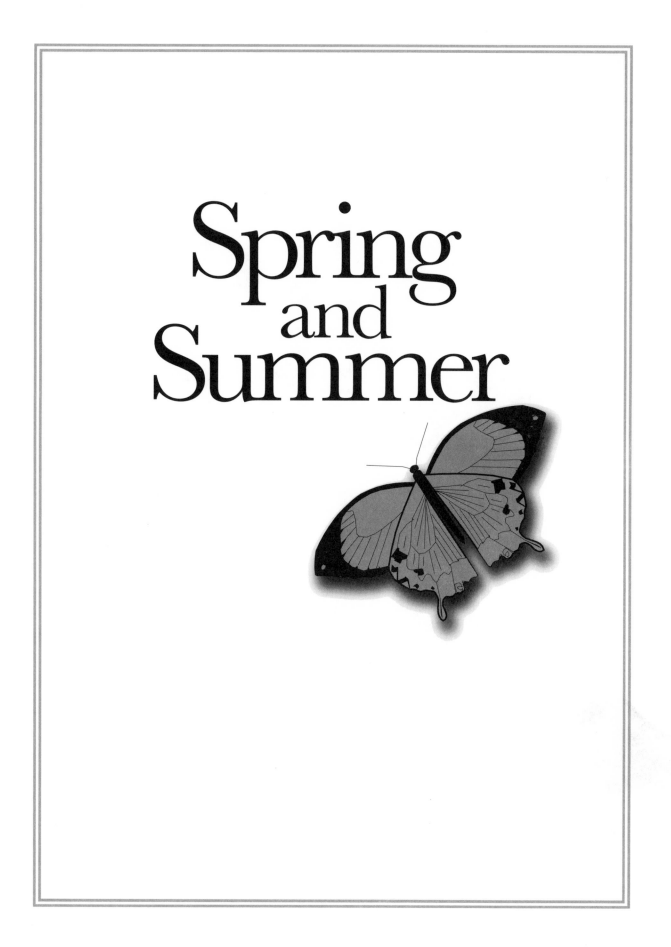

Life Can Be Beautiful

(For use especially in spring and summer or on a birthday)

Theme: It is through struggle that new life can occur for us.

Materials Needed:

1. Tape of "spring-like" instrumental music
2. Tape player
3. Large picture or symbol of a butterfly
4. Adhesive tape
5. Cup
6. Cocoon-shaped pieces of paper
7. Pencils
8. Picture of butterfly (large enough to be seen from a short distance)
9. Small pictures of butterflies or pin-on "butterflies"

Reflection

Leader: **The Lord has drawn us all together today in order to speak to each one of us. God is telling us:**

> **Look for beauty today. Draw beauty from every flower and butterfly, from everything that is new and fresh and growing. Listen for the joy in the song of the birds. Find it in those around you, especially in the children. Look at a flower until its beauty becomes part of your very soul. In the end, you will return that beauty to the world in the form of a smile, a loving word, a kind thought, a prayer, or even a tear.**

> **Listen to a bird. Take the song it sings as a message from God, our Father. Let it sink into your soul. That, too, you will return to the world.**

> **Watch a butterfly. Its struggle to emerge from its cocoon has given strength and beauty to its beautiful wings. That struggle will be given back to the world in the form of color beyond the imagination.**

> **All these are signs of new life after a cold and dreary winter season.**

Let's consider the quiet and gentleness of new life as we listen to some instrumental music.

The leader plays instrumental music for two or three minutes.

Ritual of Sharing Struggles

Leader: **Today, let us look at one particular sign of new life, of rebirth, of the breathtaking beauty of spring and summer: the butterfly.**

The butterfly moves from shriveled cocoon to beauty and gracefulness, to abundant color and the capacity to soar beyond all boundaries. And all because it persisted in its struggle to gain new life.

I'd like to tell you a story: One day a man saw a butterfly shuddering on the sidewalk, locked in a seemingly hopeless struggle to free itself from its now useless cocoon. Feeling pity, he took a pocket knife, carefully cut away the cocoon, and set the butterfly free. To his dismay, it lay on the sidewalk, convulsed weakly for a while, and died. A biologist later told him, "That was the worst thing you could have done! A butterfly needs the struggle to develop the muscles to fly. By robbing him of the struggle, you made him too weak to live."

And we realize that we too must struggle in order for new life to begin to take place in us. We are gathered here because we have lost our loved ones. The struggle we have gone through because of that has been unbearable. And yet we have not given up, or we would not be able to even come together here.

One way we can start to strengthen our muscles after our loss is to share our struggles. If we keep them locked up within us, we are never freed from the cocoons that surround us.

There are pieces of paper shaped like cocoons here for you. I invite you to take a moment and write down what you are struggling with right now (i.e., anger, depression, disbelief, etc.).

The leader distributes pieces of paper and allows two or three minutes for the participants to write while the instrumental music plays softly. After this is done, the leader asks the participants to share their "struggles" with the person beside them.

Leader: **Now please come forward and place your "struggle" in the cup on the table.**

The leader allows a moment for the participants to do this.

Leader: **Now that our struggles have been shared, let us receive a sign of new life to take home.**

The leader passes out small pictures or pins of butterflies, saying:

Receive a sign of new life!

Final Blessing

Leader: **"God speaks to us through two mediums: through other people and through nature. He reveals his love for us through the gentle eyes of a child just as easily as the ever-peaceful call of a bluebird. He knows how much we have grieved and how much we have cried. Subtly, God teaches us that:**

All: "For every tear we shed, we will laugh;
For every sadness we are burdened with,
we come to know the value of each joy;
For every loss we endure, we will be
further enriched with his peace.
For every moment we doubt his existence,
he will give us an hour, a day, a season
to see and feel that he does truly exist.

"He is there for us and has always been.
From the beginning of his time,
spring always follows the winter.
After the sorrow of our tears,
there must follow the daffodils of new life."[1]

Leader: **May we continue to struggle from the darkness of the cocoons that surround us, so that one day we can emerge into the beauty of new life. Amen.**

Life Can Be Beautiful

Theme: It is through struggle that new life can occur for us.

Reflection

Ritual of Sharing Struggles

Final Blessing

Leader: "God speaks to us through two mediums: through other people and through nature. He reveals his love for us through the gentle eyes of a child just as easily as the ever-peaceful call of a bluebird. He knows how much we have grieved and how much we have cried. Subtly, God teaches us that:

All: **"For every tear we shed, we will laugh;**
For every sadness we are burdened with,
we come to know the value of each joy;
For every loss we endure, we will be
further enriched with his peace.
For every moment we doubt his existence,
he will give us an hour, a day, a season
to see and feel that he does truly exist.

"He is there for us and has always been.
From the beginning of his time,
spring always follows the winter.
After the sorrow of our tears,
there must follow the daffodils of new life."*

Leader: May we continue to struggle from the darkness of the cocoons that surround us, so that one day we can emerge into the beauty of new life. Amen.

* Adapted from "The Sycamore Retreat," *Mortal on the Mend*, Vincent Marquis, Wallingford, CT (unpublished). Permission granted for duplication.

Signs of New Life

(For use especially in spring or summer)

Theme: New life can be found all around us.

Materials Needed:

1. Tape of instrumental music
2. Tape: "The Lilies of the Field," John Michael Talbot (see "Resources Needed," p. 11) or use the instrumental music
3. Tape player
4. (Optional) "Symbols of new life," which participants are asked to bring

Introduction

Leader: **There is a beautiful message in the Gospel of Matthew, a message of love, compassion, and hope:**

Look at the birds flying around: they don't plant or gather or store in barns—yet God, our Father takes care of them. . . . Look at how the wild flowers grow: they don't work or sew their own clothes—yet God, our Father clothes them in beauty and delight (Mt 6:24-34).

And so we say together:

All: Look at the wild flowers:
from the lifeless ground, a green shoot;
from the dry seed, a fragrant blossom.
And look at us:

It seems the Lord is inviting us to trust in his Father,
to believe that he has both the capacity and the love
to take us as we are—
wounded and scarred though we may be—
and be with us as we struggle on our journey
toward the beauty of new life.

The leader plays selected music for two or three minutes.

Gathering Ritual and Reflection

Leader: **We all need signs or symbols to help us to understand more clearly what we are trying to grasp: where we are trying to go. Look around you in this room. Is there a symbol here that says "new life" to you?**

What is that symbol? Would you share with us just why that could speak of new life for us?

Optional Symbols:

(1) Have participants bring with them a symbol of new life to share with the group (e.g., picture of baby, something they treasure, a friend).

(2) Have participants go outside and find a symbol of new life to share with the group (e.g., flower, shell, twigs, leaf).

The leader gives the participants an opportunity to share while instrumental music plays softly.

Leader: **You have shared your symbol of "new life," your gift of life, with us. Why don't we listen for a moment to what the Lord tells us as he holds each one of us in his hands and offers us new life?**

The leader pauses for a brief moment of silence.

The Lord speaks to each one of us. He tells us to seek beauty: to draw beauty from every flower and butterfly; to seek joy from the song of the birds and the color of the flowers. He tells us to drink in the beauty of the air and the water. He reminds us that suffering need not prevent our seeing the beauty around us.

If we are willing to open ourselves to the new life around us, we will find that it helps us to heal, that it reminds us of the new life awakening within us.

There are many signs of new life in the people around us, some of whom need our prayers. Let us pray together, naming those for whom we would like to pray.

The leader allows a few moments for the participants to mention their intentions.

Leader concludes:

Lord, hear our prayers.

Final Blessing

Leader: **Let us extend our hands over each other and pray that God will send each of us new hope and new life through the gifts that he is so eager to give us.**

All: May the peace and blessing
of Almighty God, Father, Son, and Holy Spirit,
descend upon us and remain with us
as we leave this place and return to our homes.

Signs of New Life

Theme: New life can be found all around us.

Introduction

Leader: And so we say together:

All: **Look at the wild flowers:**
from the lifeless ground, a green shoot;
from the dry seed, a fragrant blossom.
And look at us:
It seems the Lord is inviting us to trust in his Father,
to believe that he has both the capacity and the love
to take us as we are—
wounded and scarred though we may be—
and be with us as we struggle on our journey
toward the beauty of new life.

Gathering Ritual and Reflection

Prayer

Final Blessing

Leader: Let us extend our hands over each other and pray that God
will send each of us new hope and new life through the gifts
that he is so eager to give us.

All: **May the peace and blessing**
of Almighty God, Father, Son, and Holy Spirit,
descend upon us and remain with us
as we leave this place and return to our homes.

In Remembrance of Life Given and Nourished

(For use especially on Mother's Day, in May,
or on the birthday or anniversary of death
of a mother or grandmother)

Theme: A parent's unbounded love

Materials Needed:

1. Tape: Instrumental music or "Ave Maria" (see "Resources Needed," p. 11) or another song celebrating Mary, the Mother of God
2. Tape player
3. Vase of flowers (enough for at least one per participant)
4. List of names of deceased mothers or grandmothers of participants.
   The leader may give the participants an opportunity to list these names on a sheet of paper before the service begins, or the participants may simply say these names aloud at the appropriate point.

Introduction

Leader: **We come together to remember those who have given us the gift of life. We honor our mothers and grandmothers who gave us life and nurtured that life as they surrounded us with love. We see this in the life of Mary, the Mother of God, who sacrificed courageously for her son.**

Many were the times that she didn't understand what he was about. After losing him in the temple she exclaims: "Child, why have you treated us like this? [We] have been searching for you in great anxiety" (Luke 2:48). Then, at the wedding at Cana, Jesus tells her she shouldn't be concerned about the lack of wine: "Woman, what concern is that to you and to me?" (John 2:4). She finds it difficult to understand, yet she has an undaunted faith in her son. Many of our mothers have shown a similar faith in us.

Let us pause for a moment as we gather the memories we have of the love of our own mothers and grandmothers.

The leader plays selected music for two or three minutes.

Gathering Ritual and Reflection

Leader: In the front of the room is a vase of flowers, placed there in honor of our deceased mothers or grandmothers. I invite you to come up individually as I read their names *(or the participants may say their own mothers' or grandmothers' names)* and take a flower from the vase and then return to your place.

The leader allows enough time for the participants to go forward one by one.

Leader: Scripture is filled with stories of how God has constantly cared for his people. The New Testament recounts Jesus' acts of compassion and healing, blessing and love for those who suffer and for those who are distraught or hopeless. In a wonderful passage from Luke (Lk 12:22-28), he reminds us ". . . [not to] worry about [our] life . . ."

Jesus goes on to say: "Consider the liles how they grow: they neither toil nor spin; yet . . . Solomon in all his glory was not clothed like one of these. . . . But if God so clothes the grass of the field . . . how much more will he clothe you . . . (Luke 12:22, 27-28).

Let us for a moment "consider the lilies" *(or mention the kind of flower the participants hold).* What happened to these flowers during the past winter season? Where were they when we needed their beauty and color as we mourned the deaths of our mothers and grandmothers? They seemed to be entirely gone, for the winds and rains of the fall and the ice and snow of the winter tore at them and covered them from our view. And yet we know, because we see their beauty today, that no matter how deep our winter grieving is, spring and all its beauty and new life always follows.

Christ told us not to worry. He told his own mother the same thing after he was lost at the Temple and when her friends ran out of wine at the wedding feast. Our mothers and grandmothers may have reminded us not to worry. When we were buried in our own problems, they often found a way to remind us of the coming spring.

We hold spring flowers in our hands. We also hold memories of our mothers and grandmothers in our hearts. Those memories can begin to change our mourning into laughter, our winter into spring. As we hold those memories tenderly, as we remember what we loved best about our mothers and grandmothers, we will find that we are gradually able to move forward to new life.

Leader: Let us read together.

All: We hold in our hands the flowers
that embody new life.
We know that our mothers and grandmothers
would want us to continue on our journey
to find new life for ourselves.

Leader: **Let us take these flowers home and nurture them in remembrance of those who spent their lives nurturing us.**

Final Blessing

Leader: **Let us pray a final blessing together.**

All: And now we ask:
Lord, God, keep us in quiet and peace
as we return to our homes.
Keep us safe and turn our hearts to you
that we may be ever mindful of the unbounded love
of our mothers and grandmothers.
May your love and peace bless and console us
and gently wipe every tear from our eyes.

We ask this through Christ our Lord, and the Holy Spirit,
who together with you live forever and ever. Amen.

In Remembrance of Life Given and Nourished

Theme: A parent's unbounded love

Introduction

Gathering Ritual and Reflection

Leader: Let us read together.

All: **We hold in our hands the flowers
that embody new life.
We know that our mothers and grandmothers
would want us to continue on our journey
to find new life for ourselves.**

Final Blessing

Leader: Let us pray a final blessing together.

All: **And now we ask:
Lord, God, keep us in quiet and peace
as we return to our homes.
Keep us safe and turn our hearts to you
that we may be ever mindful of the unbounded love
of our mothers and grandmothers.
May your love and peace bless and console us
and gently wipe every tear from our eyes.**

**We ask this through Christ our Lord, and the Holy Spirit,
who together with you live forever and ever. Amen.**

What Can the Sea Teach Me?

(For use at any time)

Theme: A shell is a gift from the sea that can teach us many things during our time of suffering.

Materials Needed:

1. Tape of instrumental music evoking the sea
2. Tape: "City of God," Dan Schutte, S.J. *(Glory and Praise*, #187)—see "Resources Needed," p. 11.
3. Tape player
4. Shells (one for each participant)

Introduction

Leader: **Let us pray. Father, we come before you today in prayer. We are tired and need to be content with letting your love and understanding wash over us and heal us. Perhaps now we can be content to stop and listen to what the sea will teach us. The sea does not reward those who are too anxious, or too impatient. Patience is what the sea teaches. Patience and faith. Father, we need to be empty and open, as we wait for whatever will be our gift from the sea.**

The leader plays instrumental music for two or three minutes.

Gathering Ritual and Reflection

The leader hands one shell to each participant.

Leader: **Shells are gifts from the sea. Every beach has them, all washed up from the sea. No two are alike; each reveals different kinds of beauty to different people. Most shells are simple, bare, but beautiful. Their colors differ, yet all are whitened by a wash of salt from the sea. Look at your shell; listen to the surf that washed it up; what do you see? What do you hear?**

- **Is the shell for you just empty, because that which was in it is no longer there?**

- **Is the shell for you a beautiful piece of architecture, its lines whirling in a gentle spiral ingrained in the very fabric of its being?**

- **Does the shell remind you of the temptation to wrap protection around yourself so that nothing can harm you?**

- **Or is your shell a gift from the sea that holds infinite possibilities and dreams? Can you see it as a gift from the Creator of all shells?**

We need but also love the shell, prize it, take care of it, and know it— and that gift from the sea will become unique, treasured, and special. What does your shell, your gift from the sea, say to you today? What can it say to you in the tomorrows of your life?[2]

All: We hold our shells, our gift from the sea, in our hands.

What does the Lord tell us as he holds the gift of each one of us in his hands?

"I will be with you to the end of time. I will be with you."

Leader: **What is God saying to you particularly at this time? Take a moment to listen for his voice to you. If you are comfortable doing so, please share with the group what you feel God is telling you.**

The leader plays selected music softly and allows time for each participant to share what the shell means to him or her.

Leader: **There are many people, many beautiful gifts like these shells, in our lives. Let us pray together, naming those for whom we would like to pray.**

The leader allows a few moments for the participants to mention their intentions.

Leader concludes:

Lord, hear our prayers.

Final Blessing

All: God of love,
when you walked on the earth
you cured those who were in need of healing.
Take us by the hand now as you did to others
on so many of your journeys
and help us to rise up.
We need to walk with renewed strength and vigor.
Stretch out your hand
and touch all within us that needs to be healed.[3]

Leader: We leave now, having spent time in God's presence and in the presence of each other. Patience, faith, openness, simplicity, solitude . . . there are many things the sea has to teach us. And there are other beaches to explore; there are more shells to find. This is only a beginning. We thank the Lord for giving us the power to begin again and to journey together toward the creation of a new life. We can build for ourselves a lasting city in which we will dwell with God and those we love for all eternity.

Let us proclaim our hope for new life by singing "City of God."

All join in singing "City of God," Dan Schutte, S.J., (Glory and Praise, #187).

What Can the Sea Teach Me?

Theme: A shell is a gift from the sea that can teach us many things during our time of suffering.

Introduction

Gathering Ritual and Reflection

Leader: What does your shell, your gift from the sea, say to you to-day? What can it say to you in the tomorrows of your life?

All: **We hold our shells, our gift from the sea, in our hands.**

What does the Lord tell us as he holds the gift of each one of us in his hands?

"I will be with you to the end of time. I will be with you."

Final Blessing

All: **God of love,**
when you walked on the earth
you cured those who were in need of healing.
Take us by the hand now as you did to others
on so many of your journeys
and help us to rise up.
We need to walk with renewed strength and vigor.
Stretch out your hand
and touch all within us that needs to be healed.*

Concluding Reflection and Song

* Adapted from *Praying Our Goodbyes*, by Joyce Rupp, p. 176.

Our Father

(For use especially on Father's Day)

Theme: A father's love cannot be measured.

Materials Needed:

1. Tape: "Yahweh, the Faithful One *(Glory and Praise,* #58) or "You Are Near" *(Glory and Praise,* #59) or "Glory and Praise to Our God" *(Glory and Praise,* #17) or "Turn to Me" *(Glory and Praise,* #57)—See "Resources Needed," p. 11.
2. Tape player
3. Cup (large, chalice-type)
4. Christ candle and matches
5. Candles for participants
6. Small papers and pencils for participants

Introduction

Leader: **Whenever we reflect on the role of "father," we automatically think about strength, protection, providing, giving, caring, knowledge. Somehow we believe that if one is a father, he should know all things—and do them well. And often, that is what happens. But all of our fathers had struggles and disappointments, too. Today we remember our fathers, and we focus on the capacity of our heavenly Father to love beyond all measure.**

Let's meditate quietly on the love of God, our Father.

The leader plays selected music softly for two or three minutes.

Gathering Reflection and Ritual

Leader: **We know that Christ "loved beyond all measure" while he was on earth and that he continues to love today through the Father and the Spirit. If we were to take a cup** (leader indicates cup sitting on table) **and try to measure that love, we know the cup would overflow. So, too, the love of our Father for us.**

We know that the cup from which Christ drank included suffering. The sufferings were so great, in fact, that he asked his Father in the garden of Gethsemane, "if it were possible [to] let this cup pass from [him]"

(Matthew 26:39). **Our own fathers also faced sufferings of various kinds.**

Christ's cup of blessings was also part of his life. That cup was filled with blessings for family, friends, his ministry, a compassionate and loving personality, and a close union with, and love of, his own Father. We remember that our fathers had blessings as well as sufferings.

I invite you to think about your father's blessings for a moment. Write down a particular one you are grateful for, and then come forward and place your blessing in the cup so that we can fill it to overflowing.

As you place your blessing in the cup, please light your candle from the Christ candle while you thank your God for the gift of your father as light and life.

The leader allows several minutes for the participants to write and then come forward.

Leader: **Let us together call on our Father in heaven.**

All: Our Father, who art in heaven,
hallowed be thy name.
Thy kingdom come,
Thy will be done
on earth as it is in heaven.
Give us this day our daily bread
and forgive us our trespasses
as we forgive those who trespass against us.
And lead us not into temptation,
but deliver us from evil.
For the kingdom, the power, and the glory are yours,
now and forever. Amen.

Final Blessing

All: May the God and Father of our Lord Jesus Christ
welcome and embrace our fathers
who are with him in heaven.
And together may they continue
to love and protect and console us here on earth
until we are united.
In the Name of the Father and of the Son
and of the Holy Spirit. Amen.

Our Father

Theme: A father's love cannot be measured.

Introduction

Gathering Ritual and Reflection

Leader: Let us together call on our Father in heaven.

All: **Our Father, who art in heaven,**
hallowed be thy name.
Thy kingdom come,
Thy will be done
on earth as it is in heaven.
Give us this day our daily bread
and forgive us our trespasses
as we forgive those who trespass against us.
And lead us not into temptation,
but deliver us from evil.
For the kingdom, the power, and the glory are yours,
now and forever. Amen.

Final Blessing

All: **May the God and Father of our Lord Jesus Christ**
welcome and embrace our fathers
who are with him in heaven.
And together may they continue
to love and protect and console us here on earth
until we are united.
In the Name of the Father and of the Son
and of the Holy Spirit. Amen.

Celebration of Life

(For use especially on anniversaries or at Easter)

Theme: Eternal life is a cause for celebration.

Materials Needed:

1. Paschal candle (stands lighted in a prominent place)
2. Small candles for each participant
3. Tape: "We Remember," Marty Haugen (see "Resources Needed," p. 11) or instrumental music
4. Tape player

Before the service begins, each participant should be given a small, unlighted candle.

Introduction

Leader: **Isaiah foretold,**

> **The people who walked in darkness**
> **have seen a great light;**
> **Upon those who dwelt in the land of gloom**
> **a light has shone.**
> **You have brought them abundant joy and great**
> **rejoicing,**
> **As they rejoice before you** (Is 9:1).

The Easter Proclamation sings of mystery accomplished beyond the hope of the prophets. In the joyful announcement of the resurrection, even human suffering finds itself transformed. The fullness of joy springs from the victory of the crucified Jesus, from his pierced heart and his glorified body. This victory enlightens the darkness of our hearts and souls and gives us eternal hope in new life.

The leader plays selected music for two or three minutes and then leads the participants in reading the refrain of "We Remember" aloud as printed below.

Leader: **"We remember how you loved us to your death,**
And still we celebrate
for you are with us here.

All: "And we believe that we will see you
when you come in your glory, Lord.
We remember, we celebrate, we believe."[4]

Gathering Reflection and Ritual

Leader: **My friends, standing in the brightness of this holy light, join with me in remembering the promises God has made to us.**

If there are enough participants, the leader may divide those gathered into three groups, asking each to read one of the following verses.

All: "Consider the lilies how they grow:
they neither toil nor spin;
yet I tell you, even Solomon in all his glory
was not clothed like one of these."
(Luke 12:27)

"Consider the ravens:
they neither sow nor reap,
they have neither storehouse nor barn,
and yet God feeds them!"
(Luke 12:24)

"Blessed are the eyes that see what you see!
For I tell you that many prophets and kings
desired to see what you see, but did not see it,
and to hear what you hear, but did not hear it."
(Luke 10:23-24)

Leader: **Each one of our readings has mentioned the wonder of seeing: "Look at the wild flowers," "Look at the ravens," "How fortunate you are to see!" We celebrate today the life of someone we saw and loved—both physically and spiritually.**

I would ask that each of you approach the Paschal candle with your candles and, as you light your own candle from it, please share with the group one gift that you saw in your loved one that you would like to celebrate today.

The leader goes first, mentions something like "I saw in Jane, my mother, the gift of tenderness," lights his or her candle and returns to his or her seat. The leader then allows enough time for each participant to go forward.

Leader: **"We remember how you loved us to your death,
And still we celebrate
for you are with us here.**

All: "And we believe that we will see you
when you come in your glory, Lord.
We remember, we celebrate, we believe."[5]

Final Blessing

Leader: **We have been blessed by the gift of our loved ones.**
They have helped to make us strong, yet gentle;
wise, yet simple, restless, yet contented;
sad, yet eager to celebrate their life, here and in eternity.

All: We are grateful for the gift of our loved ones,
symbolized in the lights we hold,
lights that have been touched
by the light of the resurrected Christ.

Leader: **As we extinguish these lights now, let us take them with us to be lit**
again in our homes, and continue to celebrate life in Jesus Christ, the
light of the world.

And let us go forth in the name of the Father and of the Son and of the
Holy Spirit. Amen. Alleluia.

Celebration of Life

Theme: Eternal life is a cause for celebration.

Introduction

Leader: "We remember how you loved us to your death,
And still we celebrate
for you are with us here.

All: **"And we believe that we will see you
when you come in your glory, Lord.
We remember, we celebrate, we believe."***

Gathering Ritual and Reflection

Leader: My friends, standing in the brightness of this holy light, join
with me in remembering the promises God has made to us.

All: **"Consider the lilies how they grow:
they neither toil nor spin;
yet I tell you, even Solomon in all his glory
was not clothed like one of these flowers."**
(Luke 12:27)

**"Consider the ravens:
they neither sow nor reap.
They have neither storehouse nor barns,
And yet God feeds them!"**
(Luke 12:24)

**"Blessed are the eyes that see what you see!
For I tell you that many prophets and kings
desired to see what you see, but did not see it,
and to hear what you hear, but did not hear it."**
(Luke 10:23-24)

Leader: "We remember how you loved us to your death,
And still we celebrate
for you are with us here.

All: **"And we believe that we will see you**
when you come in your glory, Lord.
We remember, we celebrate, we believe."*

Final Blessing

Leader: We have been blessed by the gift of our loved ones.
They have helped to make us strong, yet gentle;
wise, yet simple, restless, yet contented;
sad, yet eager to celebrate their life, here and in eternity.

All: **We are grateful for the gift of our loved ones,**
symbolized in the lights we hold,
lights that have been touched
by the light of the resurrected Christ.

Leader: As we extinguish these lights now, let us take them with us
to be lit again in our homes, and continue to celebrate life in
Jesus Christ, the light of the world.

And let us go forth in the name of the Father and of the Son
and of the Holy Spirit. Amen. Alleluia.

* "We Remember," Marty Haugen (*With Open Hands* collection, © 1983 G.I.A. Publications, Inc., 7404 S. Mason Ave., Chicago, IL 60638). Permission granted for duplication.

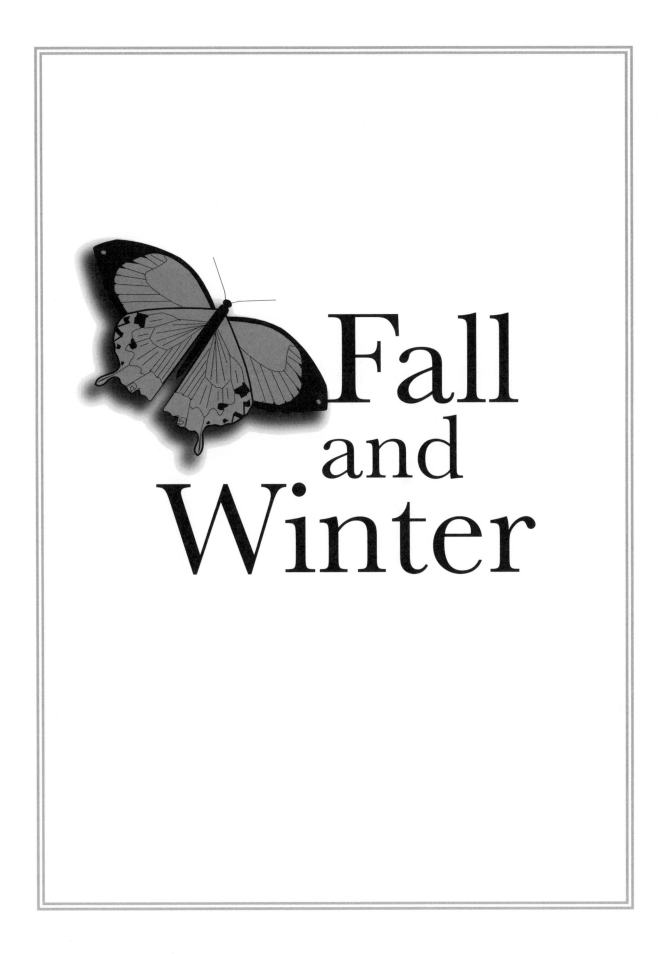

Fall
and
Winter

Thank God for the Gift of Laughter

(For use at Thanksgiving)

Theme: Laughter is a gift that can help in the healing process.

Materials Needed:

1. Tape of instrumental music
2. Tape player
3. Pencils and paper (one for each participant)

Introduction

Leader: **We know from the accounts in scripture that Jesus was a healer, a divine healer. We know also that Jesus, being fully human as well as divine, shares with us the wide range of emotions that we have: anger, fear, compassion, sorrow, joy, and yes, even the gift of laughter.**

Science now tells us that laughter and humor are an intricate part of the healing process. And so we can surmise, even though it is not written explicitly in scripture, that Jesus employed humor in his dealings with people, especially people who were in need of healing. This was perhaps just as important as compassion, tenderness, and concern.

We've all chosen our own special way to grieve the death of our loved ones, and by gathering here together we can ask the Lord to walk beside us on our journey. But even as we weep with him and ask him to weep with us, I think he also wants us to laugh with him.

Remember that it was often Jesus' joy that attracted others to him. His sufferings and death were only part of what his life was all about. If we can hold onto our sense of humor, as Jesus did, we can survive almost any emotional storm—just as Jesus did.

Gathering Ritual and Reflection

The leader gives each participant a piece of paper and pen or pencil.

Leader: **As Thanksgiving day approaches, and we anticipate being with people and celebrating the gifts that have been given us, let us begin to gather our memories of our loved ones who have died. Today, let us particularly focus on a memory of something they did or said that caused us to laugh (much like the laughing Christ in the picture on the service programs that have been given to you).**

The leader allows a moment or two of silence.

Leader: **There will be many stories shared around the table at Thanksgiving. Take a few minutes now to write down one of the stories or at least an outline about your loved one that brought you great joy and caused you to laugh.**

The leader plays instrumental music softly and allows approximately ten minutes for the participants to write at least an outline of a story.

Leader: **And now I invite you to turn to the person beside you and share that story with him or her.**

The leader allows five to ten minutes for the participants to share their stories.

Leader: **To laugh, of course, means to be joyous, to celebrate.**

Thanksgiving is certainly a time when we want to do that. Let us take our joy-filled stories to the table on Thanksgiving day and share that joy with others who will be feeling the loss of our loved one. This is a time in our lives that we need to have reminders that we can laugh, that laughter will help us to heal, that life can have its lighter moments, and that we can thank God for those moments.

Reflection

Leader: **Before we leave today, let us reflect on a story about Abraham and Sarah in the Old Testament** (Genesis 17:17; 18:13-15).

Abraham was 100 years old; his wife Sarah was 90. They both wanted a child, but did not have one. Then, God appeared to our 100-year-old Abraham and told him that his wife Sarah would give birth to a son. Abraham literally doubled over with laughter. Apparently, God was laughing with him: God told Abraham to name his son "Isaac," which in Hebrew means "God's laugh." Later, when Sarah heard a mysterious stranger give the same prophecy, she, too, laughed at the thought. This time, though, God reminded Abraham and Sarah that, even as they laughed, they should also trust. The Lord asked Abraham, "Why did Sarah laugh and say, `Can I really have a child when I am so old?' Is

anything too hard for the Lord? As I said, nine months from now I will return, and Sarah will have a son."

In due time, Sarah did give birth to a son. And she said, "God has brought me joy and laughter. Everyone who hears about it will laugh with me." And no doubt a lot of people did laugh—good, healing, healthy, joyous laughter.

Final Blessing

Leader: **May the God of Abraham and Sarah**
bless us with a spirit of joy this Thanksgiving
as we share our stories of love and laughter.

All: May this celebration be for each one of us
a reminder of the eternal celebration we will take part in
with our loved ones in heaven.

Thank God for the Gift of Laughter

Theme: Laughter is a gift that can help in the healing process.

Introduction

Gathering Ritual

Reflection

Final Blessing

Leader: May the God of Abraham and Sarah
bless us with a spirit of joy this Thanksgiving
as we share our stories of love and laughter.

All: **May this celebration be for each one of us**
a reminder of the eternal celebration we will take part in
with our loved ones in heaven.

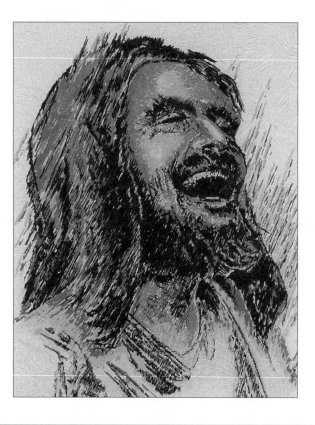

We Are Precious Gifts

(For use especially in the Christmas season)

*Theme: Even though we are suffering, we can reach out to others
and be a gift of healing.*

Materials Needed:

1. Tape of instrumental music
2. Tape player
3. Pitcher of water and bowl (placed on a table in a prominent spot)

Introduction

Leader: **Anne Morrow Lindbergh, in her *Gift From the Sea,* has described the
kind of time we have together today. She wrote,**

> **Here there is time; time to be quiet; time to work without pres-
> sure; time to think. . . . Time to look at the stars or to study a
> shell; time to see friends, to gossip, to laugh, to talk. Time, even
> not to talk. . . . Here . . . I find I can sit with a friend without
> talking, sharing the day's last sliver of pale green light of the
> horizon or the whorls in a small white shell, or the dark scar
> left in a dazzling night sky by a shooting star. Then communi-
> cation becomes communion and one is nourished as one never
> is by words.[6]**

**Let us take some time now to quiet ourselves so that we can be
nourished.**

The leader plays instrumental music for two or three minutes.

Gathering Ritual and Reflection

Leader: **Please join me in raising hands over this water to ask God's blessing.**

All: God of Creation and of Life,
pour out your blessing upon this water.
Let it be a sign of your life-giving presence and power.
As we use it in blessing, may we be filled
with your grace and strength and healing
in the name of your Son, Jesus Christ, our Lord.

Spirit of Life, though we are many,
we are one body in union with you.
We are joined to each other today
as different parts of that one body.
Help us to use our different gifts
in accordance with your grace.

Leader: **Each of us has gifts that can help others in their journeys toward healing. What gifts do you have that can help others?**

The leader allows a brief moment of silence.

I invite you to come now, one by one, and pour a small bit of water from the pitcher into the bowl. As you pour, please name one gift you have that might help others to heal from their suffering.

The leader goes first and mentions something like "compassion" or "understanding," then allows time for each participant to come forward. If desired, music may be played softly.

Leader: **You may have heard this reflection before, or perhaps read it—the author is unknown—but let's listen to it again:**

> **Persons are gifts . . . at least Jesus thought so.**
> **I am a person. Therefore, I am a gift, too.**
> **A gift for myself first of all. The Father gave myself to me.**
> **Have I ever really looked inside the wrappings?**
> **Am I afraid to?**
> **Perhaps I've never accepted the gift that I am. Could it be that there is something else inside my wrappings than what I**
>   **think there is?**
> **Maybe I've never seen the wonderful gift that I am?**
> **But could the Father's gifts be anything but beautiful?**
> **I love those gifts which those who love me give me. So why not this gift from the Father?**
> **And I am a gift to others. Am I willing to be**
> **given by the Father to others . . . a person for others?**
> **Do others have to be content with my wrappings,**
> **never really permitted to enjoy the gift of me?**
> **Every meeting of persons is an exchange of gifts.**

Leader: **There are many people, many gifts in our lives. Let us pray together, giving thanks for some of those people.**

The leader allows a few moments for the participants to mention names.

Leader concludes:

For all these, Lord, we give you thanks.

Final Blessing

All: We ask you, O Lord, as the Giver of Gifts, to bless us now.
Give us the gifts we need
to continue our journey and make new choices
that will help us to move toward new life.

The leader then asks the participants to come forward, one at a time, to dip their fingers in the bowl of water, then to return to their seats and make the sign of the cross on the forehead of the one next to them while blessing him or her in their own words.

We Are Precious Gifts

Theme: Even though we are suffering, we can reach out to others and be a gift of healing.

Introduction

Gathering Ritual and Reflection

Leader: Please join me in raising hands over this water to ask God's blessing.

All: **God of Creation and of Life,**
pour out your blessing upon this water.
Let it be a sign of your life-giving presence and power.
As we use it in blessing, may we be filled
with your grace and strength and healing
in the name of your Son, Jesus Christ, our Lord.

Spirit of Life, though we are many,
we are one body in union with you.
We are joined to each other today
as different parts of that one body.
Help us to use our different gifts
in accordance with your grace.

Final Blessing

All: **We ask you, O Lord, as the Giver of Gifts, to bless us now.**
Give us the gifts we need
to continue our journey and make new choices
that will help us to move toward new life.

The participants bless one another.

The Cross, Our Hope

(For use especially during Lent)

Theme: Hope and new life can be attained through suffering.

Materials Needed:

1. Tape: "Wood Hath Hope"(see "Resources Needed," p. 11) and "Only This I Want" *(Glory and Praise, #224)* (see "Resources Needed," p. 11) or instrumental music
2. Tape player
3. Small sticks of wood (enough for two for each participant)
4. String
5. Bible for reading gospel passages aloud.

The leader may want to ask six participants to prepare to read the following passages: (1) Luke 22:14-20, (2) Luke 22:39-46, (3) Matthew 26:47-56, (4) Luke 22:63-65, (5) John 19:25-27, and (6) Luke 23:44-46. It will make reading easier if each of these six has a bible of his or her own, with the appropriate passage marked.

Introduction

Leader: **The symbolism of the cross appears in the New Testament throughout the sayings and stories of Jesus. We are told that "those who follow him must take up their cross." By doing this, we lose our life in order to gain it. And that is exactly what happened to Christ—by losing his life, by embracing the cross, he opened up new life for us all.**

We have seen the cross all our lives. In a way, we have always known Christ crucified. Think for a moment of the image of the crucifix: Christ's head is upright, his arms are extended as if to embrace the world, and in all his suffering he is dignified and forgiving.

But many times we have said to ourselves, "What good can come from suffering?" We, too, have suffered, and we need somehow to unite ourselves with Christ in our suffering.

The leader plays selected music for two or three minutes (suggestion for this point in the service: "Wood Hath Hope").

Gathering Ritual and Reflection

Leader: **When we are feeling overwhelmed by suffering, it is helpful to look at the cross of Jesus, to hear his cry, to see his pain, and to know that he understands and sees ours.**

The leader gives each participant two sticks of wood and a length of string and directs group to tie the pieces of wood together in the form of a cross.

Leader: **Sit quietly. Hold the cross you have made in your hands.**

There are many dimensions of Christ's passion. Which of these scenes most relates to your own particular suffering?

• Sit with him in love at the Last Supper where he experiences the sadness of farewell.

The leader asks one of the the participants to read Luke 22:14-20.

• Be with him in the garden where he struggles with surrender.

The leader asks one of the the participants to read Luke 22:39-46.

• Walk with him to the place of his betrayal.

The leader asks one of the the participants to read Matthew 26:47-56.

• Hear the jeers and insults flung at him in derision.

The leader asks one of the the participants to read Luke 22:63-65.

• Stand with his mother bent in sorrow.

The leader asks one of the the participants to read John 19:25-27.

• Cry out with him in surrender to the Father.

The leader asks one of the the participants to read Luke 23:44-46.

Leader: **After this reflection, look at your own sufferings. Name them symbolically. Place them on your cross.**

The leader allows a moment or two of silence.

Leader: **And now, because we are all united in the understanding of the loss we have suffered, come forward and give your cross to someone else in the room. Symbolically, we can then carry that cross for each other as a reminder to pray for each other. As you exchange crosses, give each other a personal blessing.**

The leader plays selected music softly during the exchange of crosses and blessing (suggestion for this point in the service: "Only This I Want").

Leader: **God of hope, we unite with your son, Jesus,**
and we renew our belief in your loving power and strength.

All: Even though we see no answer to our problems,
we need not despair.
We may feel as though we are persecuted,
but we know we will never be deserted by you.
We may be knocked down, but never destroyed.
Always, wherever we may be,
we can draw strength and courage
from the life, death, and resurrection of Jesus.
In his cross is our hope
because the cross has brought us all new life.
(adapted from 2 Corinthians 4:5-12)

Final Blessing

All: May the Lord be our strength
as we struggle through our loss;
May the Lord be our vision so that we can see
how to move through this suffering;
May the Lord be our companion on our journey
through every moment of every day;
And may we always be aware that the Lord walks beside us
in order to help us carry our cross of suffering.

The Cross, Our Hope

Theme: Hope and new life can be attained through suffering.

Introduction

Gathering Ritual and Reflection

Gospel passages	Luke 22:14-20	Luke 22:63-65
(read by	Luke 22:39-46	John 19:25-27
participants)	Matthew 26:47-56	Luke 23:44-46

Leader: God of hope, we unite with your son, Jesus,
and we renew our belief in your loving power and strength.

All: **Even though we see no answer to our problems,
we need not despair.
We may feel as though we are persecuted,
but we know we will never be deserted by you.
We may be knocked down, but never destroyed.
Always, wherever we may be,
we can draw strength and courage
from the life, death, and resurrection of Jesus.
In his cross is our hope
because the cross has brought us all new life.**
(adapted from 2 Corinthians 4:5-12)

Final Blessing

All: **May the Lord be our strength
as we struggle through our loss;
May the Lord be our vision so that we can see
how to move through this suffering;
May the Lord be our companion on our journey
through every moment of every day;
And may we always be aware that the Lord walks
beside us
in order to help us carry our cross of suffering.**

Light in the Lord

(For use especially at remembrance services, on All Soul's Day,
or in the Easter season)

Theme: Those who were a light to us now live in the Lord.

Materials Needed:

1. Tape: "Light a Candle," Paul Alexander (see "Resources Needed," p. 11) or instrumental music
2. Tape player
3. Candles (one per participant)
4. Matches (the entire liturgy is by candlelight)
5. Paschal candle
6. Candelabra with five candles placed in a prominent spot

The leader may want to ask five participants to be ready to light a candle on the candelabra at the appropriate time.

This liturgy is celebrated by candlelight; artificial light should be kept low. Before service begins, the leader gives each participant a candle.

Introduction

Leader: **We come together to remember those who have been a light to us here on earth. Although they are not physically present to us, the goodness that was unique to them now shines brightly before their Lord and God.**

We remember them in a very special way today by using the very symbol that Christ used to proclaim his presence among us. "I am the light of the world," he said. Our loved ones have been light to us, and so we honor and remember them in a ceremony of light.

The leader plays selected music for two or three minutes, lighting the Paschal candle while the music plays.

All: "And I will light a candle for you.
    To shatter all the darkness and bless the times we knew.
        Like a beacon in the night.
    The flame will burn bright and guide us on our way.
        Oh today I light a candle for you.

"The seasons come and go,
    And I'm weary from the change.
I keep on moving on, you know it's not the same.
    And when I'm walking all alone
    Do you hear me call your name?
Do you hear me sing the songs we used to sing?

"You filled my life with wonder, touched me with surprise,
    Always saw that something special deep within your eyes.
      And through the good times and the bad,
    We carried on with pride.
      I hold onto the love and life we knew."[7]

Gathering Ritual and Reflection

Leader: **The book of Ecclesiastes tells us:**

    There is a season for everything under the sun,
    A time to do and a time to be done,
    A time to laugh and a time to cry?
    A time to live and a time to die (Ecclesiastes 3:1).

    Let us, the living, remember those who have touched our lives in a special way, those who have helped light our way on earth, but who now enjoy eternal light and life in heaven.

    I invite you to mention the names of those who have been a light to you.

The leader plays selected music softly as the participants mention names.

All: We light a candle in memory of those who gave us life
    and those who nurtured our life:
    our birth mothers and fathers,
    our grandparents,
    our foster parents and adoptive parents.
    We place them in the care of Mary and Joseph,
    Anna and Joachim.

First candle is lit.

Pause for a moment of silence.

    We light a candle in memory
    of those who enriched our family life:
    our brothers and sisters, aunts, and uncles and cousins.
    We place them in the care
    of all those Christ called to journey with him
    during his time on earth.

Second candle is lit.

Pause for a moment of silence.

> We light a candle in memory
> of those we were privileged to give life to:
> children who have gone before us and grandchildren;
> those who died before birth
> and those who died before they should have.
> We place them in the care of Mary and Anna and Rachel.

Third candle is lit.

Pause for a moment of silence.

> We light a candle in memory of those
> whose love enriched and gifted our lives in a special way:
> our wives and husbands, our fiances.
> We place them in the care of the apostles.

Fourth candle is lit.

Pause for a moment of silence.

> We light a candle in memory of those
> who journeyed with us in a special way,
> those who shared with us
> during our youth and adulthood:
> friends, teachers, mentors, neighbors.
> We place them in the care of St. John, Mary Magdalene,
> Zaccheus, Simon, and Joseph of Arimathea.

Fifth candle is lit.

Pause for a moment of silence.

Leader: **The light of remembrance shines before all here in this gathering.**

The leader points to candelabra and Paschal candle.

> **Let us now come forward and light our own candles from the cande-
> labra. As we do so, let us mention out loud the name of our beloved
> one and then go back to our place with our candle lit. Please remain
> standing.**

*The leader plays selected music softly. The participants come up one by one, light a
candle, mention a name, go back to their places, and remain standing with candle lit.*

Final Blessing

All: Jesus Christ is the light of the world,
         a light no darkness can overpower.
         All blessing be ours through Christ,
         the light of nations,
         the glory of Israel, for ever and ever. Amen.

Everyone blows out their candles.

Light in the Lord

(A Candlelight Service)

Theme: Those who were light to us now live in the Lord.

Introduction

All: **"And I will light a candle for you.**
       To shatter all the darkness and bless the times we
         knew.
       Like a beacon in the night.
       The flame will burn bright and guide us on our way.
       Oh today I light a candle for you.

     "The seasons come and go,
       And I'm weary from the change.
I keep on moving on, you know it's not the same.
       And when I'm walking all alone
       Do you hear me call your name?
Do you hear me sing the songs we used to sing?

     "You filled my life with wonder, touched me with surprise,
       Always saw that something special deep within your
         eyes.
       And through the good times and the bad,
We carried on with pride.
       I hold onto the love and life we knew."*

Gathering Ritual and Reflection

All: **We light a candle in memory of those who gave us life**
     and those who nurtured our life:
     our birth mothers and fathers,
     our grandparents,
     our foster parents and adoptive parents.
     We place them in the care of Mary and Joseph,
     Anna and Joachim.

First candle is lit.
Pause for a moment of silence.

We light a candle in memory
of those who enriched our family life:
our brothers and sisters, aunts, and uncles and cousins.
We place them in the care
of all those Christ called to journey with him
during his time on earth.

Second candle is lit.
Pause for a moment of silence.

We light a candle in memory
of those we were privileged to give life to:
children who have gone before us and grandchildren;
those who died before birth
and those who died before they should have.
We place them in the care of Mary and Anna and Rachel.

Third candle is lit.
Pause for a moment of silence.

We light a candle in memory of those
whose love enriched and gifted our lives in a special way:
our wives and husbands, our fiances.
We place them in the care of the apostles.

Fourth candle is lit.
Pause for a moment of silence.

We light a candle in memory of those
who journeyed with us in a special way,
those who shared with us
during our youth and adulthood:
friends, teachers, mentors, neighbors.
We place them in the care of St. John, Mary Magdalene,
Zaccheus, Simon, and Joseph of Arimathea.

Fifth candle is lit.
Pause for a moment of silence.

Final Blessing

All: **Jesus Christ is the light of the world,**

   a light no darkness can overpower.

   All blessing be ours through Christ,

   the light of nations,

   the glory of Israel, for ever and ever. Amen.

Everyone blows out their candles.

* "Light a Candle," Paul Alexander (Paul Alexander Music). Permission granted for duplication.

Winter Leads to Spring

(For use especially in winter)

Theme: We, too, can survive the winter and grow into new life.

Materials Needed:

1. Small cups filled with dirt
2. Packets of seeds (enough for 4-6 seeds for each participant)
3. Tape player
4. Tape: Instrumental music or "The Holly and the Ivy" (see "Resources Needed," p. 11)

Introduction

Leader: **The seasons have two lessons they wish to teach us: all things must pass and all things shall return. We see it over and over again as fall turns into winter, and winter turns into spring. We need to look at the lessons the seasons teach us and try to use our knowledge as we journey through winter's grief, some of us stumbling, some of us falling, some of us buried deep in the cold that our loss brings. In our grief, we have truly experienced what nature experiences each winter season: a loss of beauty, a loss of life, and a loss of growth.**

But you know, those losses are not the whole story. That's only what we see. Something happens during the fall and winter seasons that we don't see—if it didn't, spring and summer could never happen.

And so, too, even though we have experienced the loneliness and hardship of a fall and winter season, through our grief, something has been going on in us that will eventually lead not only to survival, but to growth.

The leader plays selected music for two or three minutes.

Gathering Ritual and Reflection

Leader: **We have before us on the table a small cup of dirt and packets of seeds. We know that if we plant the seeds outside, they won't grow because of the harsh weather. But we also know that if we plant them deeply within the dirt and water and nourish them within the warmth of our homes, and tenderly care for them, that even though it is winter outside, survival** and growth can occur inside. If we take care of the seeds, and are present to them each day, turning them toward the sunlight and supplying the life-giving water they need, that eventually, despite the winter weather, they will grow.

Let us each take a cup of dirt, and a packet of seeds, and take the time now, to plant those seeds.

Each participant takes a cup of dirt and plants several seeds.

Leader: There's a beautiful story called *The Tree That Survived the Winter*, written by Mary Fahey. In it, she tells us that trees survive winter after winter and lend beauty and hope summer after summer because they are able to reach out to others with their gifts of shade, strength, fruit, and beauty. Though once ravaged by winter, trees survive and can share the gifts of their newfound growth.

We, gathered here, have chosen to reach out through our pain to be with others, so that together, we can heal. The healing will never be perfect; there will always be scars. Love has the capacity to leave scars. But the scars can produce a strength and growth beyond survival.

The author in the book uses a tree; Christ used a cross made of wood; we use the inner strength God gives us to move beyond the winter seasons to the freshness and growth of spring and summer and resurrection. The growing may be difficult; indeed the grieving was and is. But that growth-journey is never made alone if we reach out to others and then allow God to walk with us.

As a symbol of walking together through this winter season of our grief, let us exchange our cups of dirt and newly planted seeds with the person next to us. Then let us go home and nourish those seeds and care for them so that in union with each other we can begin to move together beyond mere survival.

Final Blessing

Leader: Let us go forth now, remembering this:

"On the Seventh Day while he rested
God was in a quandary.
His magnificent universe
stretching resplendantly beyond mortal description
Held His new blue-green ball in its center;
there in the playground of His Heavens
and rich with life and food—

the home for His most beloved of all life.
They would have everything they need
Without further crafting by Him, save one thing:
How would they learn to Heal?

All: "In a cosmic second came His answer:
Motion.
He loved them so much
that He set the galaxies spinning—
every one of the billion times billion,
He loved them so much;
every star He sent hurling into circles of circles,
He loved them so much;
every one of the planets and moons He sent swirling,
He loved them so much;
the new sphere of their home He tilted
and with a flick of His fingers twirled it,
He loved them so much.

"He smiled liked a child with a top.
There.
It's done.
Now they will understand.

Leader: **"From that moment on,**
all the nights of humanity would pass into mornings;
all the winters would pass into springs."8

Winter Leads to Spring

Theme: We, too, can survive the winter and grow into new life.

Introduction

Gathering Ritual and Reflection

Final Blessing

Leader: Let us go forth now, remembering this:

"On the Seventh Day while he rested
God was in a quandary.
His magnificent universe
stretching resplendantly beyond mortal description
Held His new blue-green ball in its center;
there in the playground of His Heavens
and rich with life and food—
the home for His most beloved of all life.
They would have everything they need
Without further crafting by Him, save one thing:
How would they learn to Heal?

All: **"In a cosmic second came His answer:**
Motion.
He loved them so much
that He set the galaxies spinning—
every one of the billion times billion,
He loved them so much;
every star He sent hurling into circles of circles,
He loved them so much;
every one of the planets and moons He sent swirling,
He loved them so much;
the new sphere of their home He tilted
and with a flick of His fingers twirled it,
He loved them so much.

"He smiled liked a child with a top.
There.
It's done.
Now they will understand.

Leader: "From that moment on,
all the nights of humanity would pass into mornings;
all the winters would pass into springs."*

For Further Reading: *The Tree That Survived the Winter,* Mary Fahey (Mahwah, NJ: Paulist Press, 1989).

* "Passings" excerpted from *Mortal on the Mend,* by Vincent Marquis, Wallingford, CT (unpublished). Permission granted for duplication.

Holidays
and
Various
Occasions

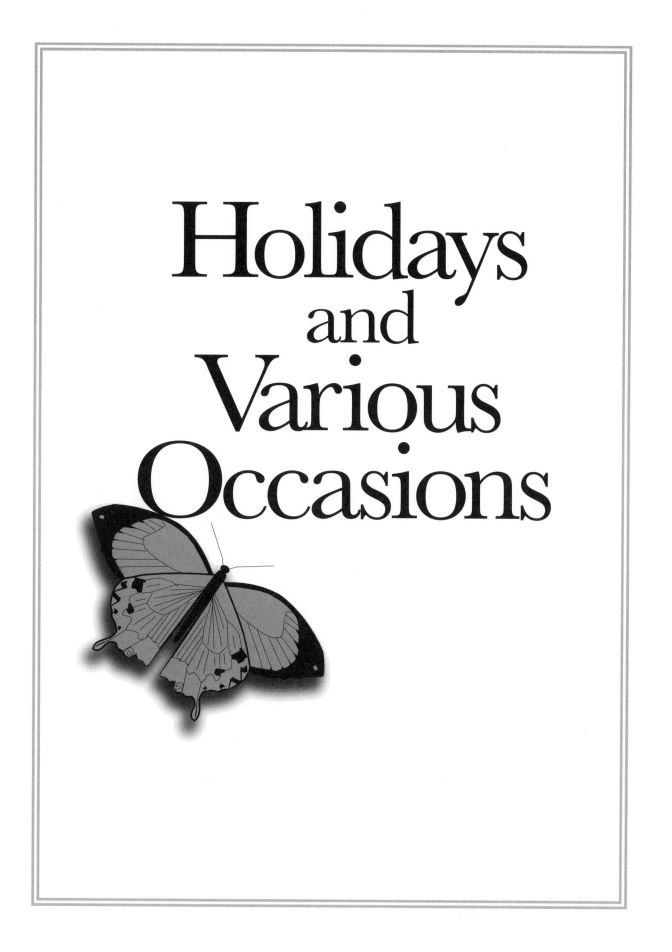

We Remember in Prayer

(For use especially on Memorial Day or an anniversary)

Theme: Prayer can be a way to remember our loved ones who have died and a means to aid us in our healing.

Materials Needed:

1. Tape: "Amazing Grace" (words in *Glory and Praise, #3*) — See "Resources Needed," p. 11.
2. Instrumental music
3. Tape player
4. Incense sticks (at least one for each participant)
5. Incense holder for leader's stick
6. A candle in a candleholder
7. Matches
8. Heat-proof plate or pan

Before the service begins, the leader lights the candle and places it in a prominent place, along with the incense sticks, incense holder, and heat-proof plate.

PSALM 23

Introduction

Leader: **Many times, we have no sense of God's presence in our grief. "Why did God allow this to happen?" we ask. "How can a good God cause such pain and suffering?" These are questions that we try to find answers to over and over again. In our most difficult times, we can't pray; we seem only to be able to cry and be angry and be in pain. Trusting in God's healing power and in his ability to intervene in our lives may be the most difficult thing we have ever tried to do.**

Because death forces us to assess our spiritual lives, the struggle with our grief can help God enter our daily existence. The hurts and wounds caused by our loss give him a chance to enter in. The healing he brings SPIRITUAL **is part of the ~~Christian~~ experience. ~~Jesus was sent by~~ God to love. He** GOD **~~showed~~ us the way to become loving. He will never abandon us as we struggle to journey through our grief.** GOD

Our God has told us over and over again that prayer is an important part of our lives. ~~The scriptures are filled with Christ's admonitions to pray, with his modeling prayer for us~~—especially at important times of change or trial. ~~He began his ministry by going off to the desert to pray~~

when the crowds pressed in on him. He took himself to a mountain, to a lake, or to a quiet place to pray. When he was about to face suffering and death, he prayed. When he was dying, he prayed. When he was saying his last earthly goodbye, he prayed. And his prayer was one of peace. In the practice of his own life, Jesus showed us that prayer is an intricate part of life and death, and that prayer can bring us peace.

Let us listen to what the Lord offers to us when we find it difficult to pray:

The leader plays "Amazing Grace" or leads the participants in reading the words of this hymn aloud.

Gathering Ritual and Reflection

Leader: **The experience of losing a loved one in death tears us quickly and forever from a life-nourishing relationship. This wrenching process leaves a deep, painful wound that we think will never heal. We soon realize that we are going to have to work hard at facing what has happened to us in order to grieve the loss we have experienced. We must acknowledge our pain and struggle through it before any kind of healing can take place. That will hurt, and there will be a scar, no matter how hard we try to cover our wound over. What we need to begin to discover are ways that will help in that healing process.**

Certainly one of those ways can be acknowledging our loss in the very core of our being—that quiet space, that place of depth and meaning where God dwells. In that place we can connect with God in a healing way, we can find help as we say these painful goodbyes.

There are many forms prayer can take during this difficult time in our lives. We may seek others to join us in vocal prayer; we may attend religious services; we may wish to be alone in prayer, to sit and wait and listen. Whatever form it takes, prayer can be a way of remembering our loved ones and helping us to continue on our healing journey.

Let us pray to God, this day, using an ancient symbolic ritual that has been a part of the church's prayer for centuries.

The leader plays instrumental music softly, lights an incense stick, and waits for the smoke to begin to rise.

Leader: **Please join me in praying Psalm 141.**

All: I call upon you, O Lord;
    come quickly to me;
give ear to my voice
    when I call to you.

Let my prayer be counted as
    incense before you,
and the lifting up of my hands
    as an evening sacrifice."
        (Ps 141:1-2)

Instrumental music continues.

Leader: **We are all parts of the one body of ~~Christ~~. To symbolize our unity in ~~Christ, I~~ ask each of you to come forward ~~and light an incense stick from the candle that is burning.~~** *PICK UP A FLAG OF REMEMBRANCE*

The leader allows time for each participant to light his or her stick from the candle and return to his or her place, holding the burning stick.

All: In memory of my loved one __(name)___,
I pray, dear God:
Let my prayer be counted as
    incense before you,
and the lifting up of my hands
    as an evening sacrifice.
        (Ps 141:1-2)

Final Blessing

Leader: **Let us recite together the "Serenity Prayer."**

All: God grant me the serenity
to accept the things I cannot change,
the courage to change the things I can,
and the wisdom to know the difference.
Living one day at a time,
enjoying one moment at a time;
accepting hardship as a pathway to peace;
taking, as Jesus did,
this sinful world as it is,
not as I would have it;
trusting that you will make all things right
if I surrender to your will;
so that I may be reasonably happy in this life
and supremely happy with you forever in the next.
Amen.

All extinguish incense sticks, or still-burning incense sticks may be placed on the plate at the front.

We Remember in Prayer

Theme: Prayer can be a way to remember our loved ones who have died and a means to aid us in our healing.

Introduction

Gathering Ritual and Reflection

Leader: Please join me in praying Psalm 141.

All:

I call upon you, O Lord;
    come quickly to me;
give ear to my voice
    when I call to you.

Let my prayer be counted as
    incense before you,
and the lifting up of my hands
    as an evening sacrifice."
        (Ps 141:1-2)

All:

In memory of my loved one, __(name)___,
I pray, dear God:
Let my prayer be counted as
    incense before you,
and the lifting up of my hands
    as an evening sacrifice.
        (Ps 141:1-2)

Final Blessing

Leader: Let us recite together the "Serenity Prayer."

All:

God grant me the serenity
to accept the things I cannot change,
the courage to change the things I can,
and the wisdom to know the difference.

Living one day at a time,
enjoying one moment at a time;
accepting hardship as a pathway to peace;
taking, as Jesus did,
this sinful world as it is,
not as I would have it;
trusting that you will make all things right
if I surrender to your will;
so that I may be reasonably happy in this life
and supremely happy with you forever in the next.
Amen.

All extinguish incense sticks, or still-burning incense sticks may be placed on the plate at the front.

Letting Go

(For use at any time)

*Theme: We need to let go of the pain and emotions that bind us,
so that God can work in our lives.*

Materials Needed:

1. Tape: "All That We Have" *(Glory and Praise, #82)* (see "Resources Needed," p. 11) or instrumental music
2. Tape player
3. Pencils and small slips of paper
4. A heat-proof plate with a candle (in a candleholder) in the center
5. Matches

Introduction

Leader: **The process of letting go is painful. We tend to think that we can be in complete control of our lives. But in reality, especially as we experience the loss of someone we love dearly, bad things do happen to good people. And we realize very clearly that these are things we can't control.**

It is in the letting go of that control and turning our lives over to God, that we can have the strength to say good-bye to one dream and begin to design another. Letting go and letting God become involved can help us to design that new dream. We will never be able to replace the old dream, but the new ones can be a powerful force in our lives.

The leader plays selected music for two or three minutes.

Gathering Ritual and Reflection

Leader: **A very important aspect of our journey toward healing after the loss of our loved one is "letting go." We see this process all around us, especially in nature.**

The seasons are all about that. Follow a tree throughout summer, fall, winter, and spring. The beautiful, rich, and full tree that stands so majestically in summer begins to shed its leaves during the fall until it stands stark and gaunt, vulnerable to the snow and winds of a harsh winter. The tree has let go of its life, but we are continually surprised as each spring unfolds to see new beauty, new strength, and new life in

that tree. It is in the letting go that the tree can eventually be open to the promise of new life.

Consider these images:

You are a small child taking your first steps away from your mom or dad . . .

Today is your first day of school, and you've been left at school for the first time . . .

You have a wonderful balloon you bought at a carnival that has become untied from your wrist and now you can barely see it as it goes higher and higher in the sky . . .

In all these images, a "letting-go" has taken place. Is that all bad? Or can "letting go" move us toward a desired end: independence, knowledge, beauty, new horizons?

Let's look for a minute at the physical side of letting go.

Please clench your fists as hard as you can . . .

Now relax your fists allowing your hands to open palms up . . .

Try it once again

How did that feel? *Pause for a moment.* Did you feel a release of tension at all? When you hold tight, only the letting go can ease the tightness, the pain, the loneliness of being closed in.

What are the feelings and thoughts you are holding onto? Which feelings and thoughts are getting in the way of you moving on in your life? For each of us they will be different. We each have different ways of getting in touch with them and different timetables in determining how and when to let go.

The emotions most likely to be in that clenched fist are anger, frustration, worry, loneliness, sadness, fear of the unknown—all feelings that have touched us over and over again. Recognizing that we have all those emotions bottled up inside us is our first step in moving toward healing.

But how do you know when it is appropriate to let go? How do you know when it's time to move on? *Pause for a moment.* When the particular emotion I'm experiencing impedes my functioning or is keeping me depressed or angry, not allowing me to see any joy, then it's time to let go.

Letting go means giving up control, but it also requires being gentle with myself. St. Peter advised his friends "to leave all your worries with

God, because he cares for you." Sometimes it's impossible to do this on our own—it's necessary to have a trusted friend, counselor, spiritual advisor to be with us to support us in that process of letting go.

Letting go at times can be like the freedom of a balloon or kite, or as painful as being in the garden of Gethsemane. But whether we experience freedom or pain, the letting go can bring us healing and new life.

Let us each take a piece of paper and write on it an emotion or a fear we have on this journey we are traveling after the death of our loved one.

The leader plays selected music softly and allows the participants time for writing. The leader then lights a candle in the middle of a heat-proof plate.

Now let us bring these slips of paper forward and allow them to be swallowed up by this flame. As we do so, we remember the task we have of letting go.

Music continues. The leader lights the candle and then lights a corner of her or his slip of paper and drops it immediately onto the plate. The participants are given time to do the same with their paper.

Final Blessing

Leader: **"If we let go and let God do his work, he will always be there for us, whether we feel his arms, or his voice, or something in nature that attracts us during one of his glorious seasons. Some leaf or limb or stream or sea may come up behind us one day and tap us on the shoulder, and whisper to us that if we let go and let God work in our lives:**

All: "Spring will come
All for the sake of his love;
All in His grand design;
All in a heartbeat of God."[9]

Leader: **Let us extend to each other God's peace as we continue to let go and journey toward new life.**

All: Amen.

Everyone exchanges greetings.

Letting Go

Theme: We need to let go of the pain and emotions that bind us, so that God can work in our lives.

Introduction

Gathering Ritual and Reflection

Final Blessing

Leader: If we let go and let God do his work, he will always be there for us, whether we feel his arms, or his voice, or something in nature that attracts us during one of his glorious seasons. Some leaf or limb or stream or sea may come up behind us one day and tap us on the shoulder, and whisper to us that "if we let go and let God work in our lives:

All: **"Spring will come**
All for the sake of his love;
All in His grand design;
All in a heartbeat of God."*

Leader: Let us extend to each other God's peace as we continue to let go and journey toward new life.

All: **Amen.**

Everyone exhanges greetings.

* Excerpted from *Mortal on the Mend,* by Vincent Marquis, Wallingford, CT (unpublished). Permission granted for duplication.

Pearls of Great Price

(For use especially on an anniversary)

Theme: We, and our loved ones, are most precious in the eyes of the Lord.

Materials Needed:

1. Tape: "Earthen Vessels" *(Glory and Praise, #13)*, "On Eagle's Wings" *(Glory and Praise, #126)* (see "Resources Needed," p. 11) or instrumental music
2. Tape player
3. Picture of a pearl or a string of pearls

The participants are asked beforehand to bring a picture of their deceased loved one with them.

Introduction

Leader: **As we approach the ~~anniversary~~ of the death of our loved one, we are filled with many different emotions. ~~On one hand, we are dreading the actual date of the anniversary; we are conscious that a year or a number of years have now passed since an extremely sad day in our lives—a day that cannot be taken back.~~** *[handwritten: REMEMBRANCE /LIFE AND] [handwritten: WE TAKE TIME TO REMEMBER]*
~~On the other hand, this anniversary is an opportunity for us~~ to celebrate in a special way the lives of those we have loved who have gone before us. *[handwritten: AND] [handwritten: ALL]*

Let us take the time today to celebrate ~~their~~ precious lives in a ceremony of remembrance.

The leader plays selected music for two or three minutes.

Gathering Ritual and Reflection

As music plays, the leader asks the participants to place the picture of their loved one that they have brought with them on the table set up in front of the room. Already on the table is a picture of a pearl or a string of pearls.

Leader: **You have just placed on the table a picture of the one you hold so dear to your heart. On the table also is a (picture of a pearl/string of pearls), which symbolizes something precious, something rare, something not easily found or attained.**

Let me tell you a story of how pearls are made. A rough bit of sand or a tiny rock fragment invades an oyster's shell as it rests at the bottom of the sea. This hurts, and the oyster tries very hard to push it out. It struggles to eject this foreign object, twisting and turning in every direction, all to no avail. The tiny invader remains. Finally, the oyster gives up in despair, determined to live with the discomfort. Then two things happen. After a while, the pain seems easier to bear; and then a crystal fluid begins to coat the tiny rock fragment or piece of sand that has invaded the shell. Gradually, a round, smooth cover develops around the fragment that grows larger and richer in color every day. While the oyster pays no more attention to what is going on within its heart, the ugly intruder is beginning to grow into a beautiful, precious pearl.

Similar things sometime happen in the life of humans. Sometimes an individual is quite ordinary and unremarkable, one who would not particularly stand out in a crowd as an exceptional person. Then adversity comes, like the death of a loved one, followed by a period of anguish over that death.

But unexpected depth and beauty can come from ordinary individuals like you and me. A faith arises within us that enables us to accept and struggle through our grief and ask God's help in bearing it. It is then, at the moment we let go of our struggling, that we begin to realize that as long as we have God with us, we need not struggle alone.

Your loved ones are pearls of great price to you, there is no doubt about that. But never forget that you, too, are precious—most especially to your God. With his help, you have been able to rise above the unlovely happenings of each day. And you have continued your struggle through your grief to the point where you can celebrate the precious life of your loved one on this anniversary.

One of the most helpful ways we have of continuing to grow after the death of a loved one is to constantly remember them, as we are doing this day. Let us join together in a litany of remembrances, calling to mind those whom we hold most precious in our eyes, our pearls of great price.

The leader plays selected music softly during the following litany.

Leader: **"In the rising of the sun and its going down,**

Participants: we remember them.

Leader: **In the blowing of the wind and in the chill of winter,**

Participants: we remember them.

Leader:	**In the opening of buds and in the rebirth of spring,**
Participants:	we remember them.
Leader:	**In the blueness of the sky and the warmth of summer,**
Participants:	we remember them.
Leader:	**In the rustling of leaves and in the beauty of autumn,**
Participants:	we remember them.
Leader:	**In the beginning of the year and when it ends,**
Participants:	we remember them.
Leader:	**When we are weary and in need of strength,**
Participants:	we remember them.
Leader:	**When we are lost and sick at heart,**
Participants:	we remember them.
Leader:	**When we have joys we yearn to share,**
Participants:	we remember them.
Leader:	**So long as we live, they too shall live,**
Participants:	for they are now a part of us, as we remember them."[10]
Leader:	~~**Please return now to take back with you the picture you have brought.**~~

The leader allows a few minutes for the participants to retrieve their pictures.

Leader:	**I invite you to turn to the person beside you, share the picture of your loved one, and tell them why you found him or her so precious in your life.**

The leader allows several minutes for all participants to share.

CLOSING: PRAYER OF BLESSINGS ⟶

Final Blessing

Leader:	**May we always remember that we, as well as our loved ones, are "pearls of great price" in the eyes of the Lord.**
All:	May he continue to bless us and walk with us as we struggle through each day. And may we pledge to each other assembled here our continued prayers. In the name of the Father and of the Son and of the Holy Spirit. Amen.

Pearls of Great Price

*Theme: We, and our loved ones, are most precious
in the eyes of the Lord.*

Introduction

Gathering Ritual and Reflection

Leader: "In the rising of the sun and its going down,

Participants: **we remember them.**

Leader: In the blowing of the wind and in the chill of winter,

Participants: **we remember them.**

Leader: In the opening of buds and in the rebirth of spring,

Participants: **we remember them.**

Leader: In the blueness of the sky and the warmth of summer,

Participants: **we remember them.**

Leader: In the rustling of leaves and in the beauty of autumn,

Participants: **we remember them.**

Leader: In the beginning of the year and when it ends,

Participants: **we remember them.**

Leader: When we are weary and in need of strength,

Participants: **we remember them.**

Leader: When we are lost and sick at heart,

Participants: **we remember them.**

Leader: When we have joys we yearn to share,

Participants: **we remember them.**

Leader: So long as we live, they too shall live,

Participants: **for they are now a part of us, as we remember them."***

Final Blessing

Leader: May we always remember that we, as well as our loved
             ones, are "pearls of great price" in the eyes of the Lord.

All: **May he continue to bless us and walk with us
             as we struggle through each day.
             And may we pledge to each other assembled here
             our continued prayers.
             In the name of the Father and of the Son and of the
             Holy Spirit. Amen.**

* Excerpted from *Gates of Prayer* (Reformed Jewish Prayerbook), p. 552. Permission
granted for duplication.

Like a Rock

(For use especially on an anniversary)

*Theme: It is in reaching out to others that we gain new strength
on our journey through grief.*

Materials Needed:

1. Tape: "On Eagle's Wings" *(Glory and Praise, #126)* (see "Resources Needed," p. 11)
   or instrumental music
2. Tape player
3. Stones (large enough to write on, one for each participant)
4. Colored markers
5. Bible (with a marker at Psalm 91)

Introduction

Leader: **There are a number of references to stones and rocks in scripture. Usually, they are described as symbols of strength and endurance:**

> **The stone that the builders rejected**
> **has become the cornerstone;**
> **this was the Lord's doing and it is**
> **amazing in our eyes.** (Mark 12:10-11)
> **and**
> **. . . You are Peter and on this rock**
> **I will build my church.** (Matthew 16:18)

A rock is strong and hard. It can be chipped, but is seldom broken. If I am "like a rock," very little can shake me; I am strong and my foundation is solid.

When I experience the death of a loved one, the very core of me, my foundation, is shaken. I allow the floods and rivers of doubt, and fear of loneliness and despair, rage against me. What must I do to regain my strength and trust in the Lord?

Let us listen to the words of the Psalmist.

The leader plays "On Eagle's Wings" (Glory and Praise, #126) or reads Psalm 91.

Gathering Ritual and Reflection

Leader: In the first chapter of the gospel of Luke, there is a story that concerns a journey. I'm sure you're familiar with Mary's journey to visit her cousin Elizabeth, after she was told by the angel that she was to be the mother of God. The gospel story tells us that "Mary set out and went with haste to a Judean town in the hill country where she entered the house of Zechariah and greeted Elizabeth . . ." (Lk 1:39).

What does the passage mean to us in our lives, lives that have been filled with struggle because of the loss we've gone through?

"Mary set out . . . " the story tells us.

Mary, who perhaps was fourteen or fifteen years old, has just been told by a messenger from God that life as she knew it—simple, carefree, probably sheltered—has suddenly been changed. In fact, life as she knew it is no more. This young girl who is not married is to become a mother, and she can't even name the father—for the angel's message had no name to give her but "spirit." And so, in the course of a very short conversation with a heavenly being, Mary's hopes and desires are shattered and changed, and she is faced with beginning a new life based solely on her faith. In a moment, Mary has lost what was indeed precious to her: her youth, the respect of the people in her town, and very likely, the understanding of the man she had hoped to marry. In this moment, Mary has lost what she has been dreaming of all her young life, and she is left confused and very vulnerable.

To those of us who have lost the person we so dearly loved, Mary's loss becomes an understandable reality. We, too, have been confused, left now without our dreams, holding tightly to the remembrances we had, reluctant to move beyond them.

But, we need to do as Mary did—to "set out." We need to walk and struggle on our journey, because shattered dreams need to be mended and new ones need to be dreamed again.

We are told in our gospel story that as soon as Mary's cousin heard her greeting, she was filled with God's presence. Mary had struggled on that difficult journey to visit her cousin and to share the miracle of the new life that was pulsating within her.

Like Mary, we did not seek out the loss we experienced. Indeed, we probably never thought it would occur. And, like Mary, we face a journey that will be long and dusty, that will take us through difficult hill country. But, we are also like Mary in another way: because of the losses we've suffered, we have the capacity to carry God's presence with us.

Some days we don't feel that. Some days, God feels far, far away. But, just as in the story of "Footprints," it's when we can't feel or see God's presence, in those very hard and dark times that we feel depressed and abandoned, when we don't see that God is journeying with us, that we can be assured he can and does carry us and is within us.

Mary had to share the presence that she carried with her on her journey. There was, in a way, no choice for her but to reach out. If she did not, it would be too painful to face these unexpected new challenges; it would be impossible to find in them a growth in faith, a chance to produce and be a part of a new life.

If we, too, can learn how to work with our grief and to reach out to others, our grief can lead to a newness and a strength that we cannot possibly comprehend now. We can gain this strength, as Mary did, from the struggle, and become "like a rock," strong and firm, able to withstand the sorrows that constantly engulf us.

And if we reach out to others in our struggle, as Mary did, our strength will only increase and eventually become a source of peace for us.

All: Rocks are a symbol of strength to us.
         They remind us that if we work at moving through our grief,
         we too, can be strong,
         especially where we find ourselves most vulnerable.

Leader: I invite you to take a stone and a marker and write on one side of that stone one particular gift you feel you need in order to help strengthen you for the journey that lies before you. It might be the gift of patience or peace or strength itself, or tears to release emotions, or something else. On the other side, please write your first name. Also feel free to decorate your stone further if you would like.

Soft music is played while the participants each pick up a stone and follow the directions above.

Leader: A very big part of the healing process—a way we can begin to build up one strength—is to reach out to others who are in pain also. It is in the reaching out that shared pain becomes easier to bear.

         I invite each of you to turn to the person beside you and exchange your rocks. In this exchange, please ask that person to pray that you receive the gift you feel you need to continue in this journey you have begun. Remember, as we pray for each other, we are continually reminded that we never journey alone.

The leader allows a moment for the participants to follow these directions.

Final Blessing

Leader: **We all have new experiences ahead of us. We have new worlds to explore, new feelings to feel, new relationships to grow into (even though they will never be the same as the relationship we had at one time with the person we loved who has died). In this process of trying to strengthen ourselves, we can be assured that we will find these new opportunities.**

All: It won't come easily; it won't come quickly.
But it will come if we continue to work at our grief.
We must remember that we are not walking this journey alone.
We can all work together to gather strength in our time of need.

Leader: **And so let us join hands, and in a spirit of prayer and love, bless each other.**

All: May the love of God
and the peace of the Lord Jesus Christ
strengthen, bless, and console us,
and gently wipe every tear from our eyes.
In the name of the Father and of the Son and of the Holy Spirit. Amen.

Like A Rock

Theme: It is in reaching out to others that we gain new strength on our journey through grief.

Introduction

Gathering Ritual and Reflection

Leader: . . . And if we reach out to others in our struggle, as Mary did, our strength will only increase and eventually become a source of peace for us.

All: **Rocks are a symbol of strength to us.**
They remind us that if we work at moving through our grief,
we too, can be strong,
especially where we find ourselves most vulnerable.

Final Blessing

Leader: We all have new experiences ahead of us. We have new worlds to explore, new feelings to feel, new relationships to grow into (even though they will never be the same as the relationship we had at one time with the person we loved who has died). In this process of trying to strengthen ourselves, we can be assured that we will find these new opportunities.

All: **It won't come easily; it won't come quickly.**
But it will come if we continue to work at our grief.
We must remember that we are not walking this journey alone.
We can all work together to gather strength in our time of need.

Leader: And so let us join hands, and in a spirit of prayer and love, bless each other.

All: **May the love of God**
and the peace of the Lord Jesus Christ
strengthen, bless, and console us,
and gently wipe every tear from our eyes.
In the name of the Father and of the Son and of the Holy Spirit.
Amen.

The Choice Is the Difference

(For marking events such as moving, going on vacation,
changing jobs, or facing the unknown)

*Theme: Choosing to continue on our journey
toward healing can make a difference.*

Materials Needed:

1. Tape: "The Path of Life," David Haas (see "Resources Needed," p. 11) or "Be Not Afraid" *(Glory and Praise, #8)*
2. Tape player
3. Footprints (paper cutouts for all participants)
4. Christ candle and matches
5. Small candles (one for each participant)

Introduction

Leader: **We have been on a difficult journey since our loved one has died. We know that many times it has been almost impossible to place one foot in front of the other. And yet we have continued to journey; in fact, those very feet that have been so hard to lift and propel forward have led us to this remembrance service today.**

Let us pause a minute and reflect on what has gotten us this far.

The leader plays selected music for two or three minutes.

Leader: **Let us read together.**

All: Wisdom delivered from tribulations
those who served her. . . .
She guided him on straight paths.
She showed him the kingdom of God.
She prospered him in his labors
and increased the fruit of his toil. . . .
She conducted them by a wondrous road
and became a shelter for them by day
and a starry flame by night (Wisdom 10:9-10, 17).

Gathering Ritual and Reflection

Leader: **When someone dies, we are given a choice between two roads—one that will help us to face the death and begin to move on our grief journey, and the other that leaves us standing still, choosing not to face what has happened.**

Robert Frost, in his poem "The Road Not Taken," depicts his questioning when faced with a decision:

> **Two roads diverged in a wood, and I—**
> **I took the one less traveled by,**
> **And that has made all the difference.**

Our grief journey is indeed a road "less traveled." It is not an easy one. But if we make a deliberate choice to travel it, that can make all the difference in the world.

Let us, symbolically, choose to continue this difficult journey. You have some cutouts of footsteps. I invite you to write on those footsteps all those things you feel you will need to continue on your journey of grief.

For instance, there are several things that I feel I need to continue: *(Leader mentions three or four things such as "friends," "a push from God," "a good support group.")* **Let's take a moment to write these things down on our footsteps.**

The leader allows a few minutes for the participants to write their answers.

Leader: **Let us place those needs before the Christ candle, and before we return to our places, light our own candles from the light and life of Christ.**

The leader goes first, and then allows time for the participants to place cut-outs in front of candle, light their own candle, and return to their places.

Leader: **God, our Father, we have acknowledged to you the needs we have as we continue our difficult journey.**

All: We ask you now to accept the names of our loved ones,
to hold them dear to you,
and to allow the memory of them
to accompany us during this time.

Leader: **Let us name aloud the loved ones we are remembering.**

The leader allows a few moments for the participants to follow these directions.

Final Blessing

Leader: **We have asked the Lord to hear our needs and to keep before and alongside of us the memory of our loved ones. And now, we ask together:**

All: God be in my head and in my understanding;
God be in my eyes that I may see your will;
God be in my thoughts as I remember my loved ones;
God be in my feet and my will as I journey toward eternal life with you.
Amen.

The Choice Is the Difference

*Theme: Choosing to continue on our journey
toward healing can make a difference.*

Introduction

Leader: Let us read together.

All: **Wisdom delivered from tribulations
those who served her. . . .
She guided him on straight paths.
She showed him the kingdom of God.
She prospered him in his labors
and increased the fruit of his toil. . . .
She conducted them by a wondrous road
and became a shelter for them by day
and a starry flame by night** (Wisdom 10:9-10, 17).

Gathering Ritual and Reflection

Leader: God, our Father, we have acknowledged to you the needs we
have as we continue our difficult journey.

All: **We ask you now to accept the names of our loved ones,
to hold them dear to you,
and to allow the memory of them
to accompany us during this time.**

Final Blessing

Leader: We have asked the Lord to hear our needs and to keep before
and alongside of us the memory of our loved ones. And now,
we ask together:

All: **God be in my head and in my understanding;
God be in my eyes that I may see your will;
God be in my thoughts as I remember my loved ones;
God be in my feet and my will as I journey toward eternal
life with you.
Amen.**

We Remember the Beginning

(For use on a birthday)

Theme: Celebration of the anniversary of the day of birth.

Materials Needed:

1. Tape of instrumental music
2. Tape: "Earthen Vessels" *(Glory and Praise, #13)* (see "Resources Needed," p. 11) or the instrumental music may be used
3. Tape player
4. Christ candle and matches
5. Small candles (one for each participant)
6. Bible

Introduction

Leader: **In the story of the birth of John the Baptist, Jesus' cousin, we are told that the neighbors and relatives were amazed that Elizabeth—who was barren and elderly—and her husband Zachariah were to give birth to a child. They could not understand God's ways and exclaimed when they heard of the birth, "What then will this child become?" (Luke 1:66).**

We know the story and what indeed did become of John. His privileged place in life was to prepare the way for his Lord. An awesome task to accomplish!

Each one of us at our birth is as unique as John the Baptist, and each one of us has a privileged place in life, a particular mission to either begin or accomplish.

We are here today to celebrate the anniversary of other births. It is, indeed, a time to take part in a celebration of the lives we treasure so dearly.

The leader plays selected music for two or three minutes.

Gathering Ritual and Reflection

Leader: **What does light mean to us?**
Listen to what the prophet Isaiah says:

I am the Lord, I have called you in righteousness,
I have taken you by the hand and kept you;
I have given you as a covenant to the people,
a light to the nations,
to open the eyes that are blind,
to bring out the prisoners from the dungeon,
from the prison those who sit in darkness (Is 42:6-7).

God can change the darkness into light by his presence. If we let that presence be a part of us, we can see in the darkness and need not be afraid. Somehow, light disperses the darkness and brings joy.

We light candles to celebrate—especially to celebrate birth. And it is the nature of celebration to have others join in and be part of it. We'll do that now as we remember the beginnings of our loved ones.

Let us pray.

All: Father, we share in the light of your glory
through your son, the light of the world.
May this fire, symbolic of Christ,
inflame us with new hope.
Purify our minds and hearts
with the lighting of this Christ candle
and bring us one day to the feast of eternal light.
We ask this through Christ our Lord. Amen.

The leader lights the Christ candle.

Leader: I invite you to take your own candle and come forward individually to take light from Christ's light. As you do so, please mention the name of your loved one whose birth we are remembering here.

Instrumental music is played as each participant comes forward.

Leader: Each candle you hold is symbolic of the light of Christ. It is a flame divided, but undimmed. In fact, it shines brighter in its division.

Gift-giving is part of every birth celebration. I ask you to turn to the person beside you and exchange your gift, your light, your candle with him or her.

The leader allows several minutes for the participants to share with each other.

Leader: Each one of us may now carry the light of Christ in remembrance of another, with us. In time of darkness or of suffering we will remember to light this particular candle and remember the one who gave it to us and the life of the one whom we celebrate.

Final Blessing

All: Lord God, we thank you for the gift of our loved ones
whose births we celebrate today.
They have, indeed, been reborn in you.
We ask you, in the beauty of these candles,
to keep us in quiet and in peace,
to keep us safe and turn our hearts to you
so that we may ourselves be light for our world.
Amen.

We Remember the Beginning

Theme: Celebration of the anniversary of the day of birth.

Introduction

Gathering Reflection and Ritual

Leader: Let us pray.

All: **Father, we share in the light of your glory**
through your son, the light of the world.
May this fire, symbolic of Christ,
inflame us with new hope.
Purify our minds and hearts
with the lighting of this Christ candle
and bring us one day to the feast of eternal light.
We ask this through Christ our Lord. Amen.

Leader: Each one of us may now carry the light of Christ in remembrance of another, with us. In time of darkness or of suffering we will remember to light this particular candle and remember the one who gave it to us and the life of the one whom we celebrate.

Final Blessing

All: **Lord God, we thank you for the gift of our loved ones**
whose births we celebrate today.
They have, indeed, been reborn in you.
We ask you, in the beauty of these candles,
to keep us in quiet and in peace,
to keep us safe and turn our hearts to you
so that we may ourselves be light for our world.
Amen.

Let Our Clay Be Moist

(For use at any time)

Theme: Our suffering can allow the Lord to mold our lives into something new.

Materials Needed:

1. Tape of instrumental music
2. Tape player
3. Clay (enough for a small piece for each participant)

Before the service begins, the leader should ask three participants to serve as readers during the service.

Introduction

Leader: **We do not shape God; God shapes us. If we are the work of God, we need to await the hand of the artist who does all things in due season. Let us offer him our hearts, soft and tractable, and keep the form in which the artist has fashioned us. As St. Irenaeus said, "Let your clay be moist, lest you grow hard and lose the imprint of his fingers."**

The leader plays instrumental music for two or three minutes.

Gathering Ritual and Reflection

Reader 1:   The Lord said to me, "Go down to the potter's house, where I will give you my message." So I went there and saw the potter working as his wheel. Whenever a piece of pottery turned out imperfectly, he would take the clay and make it into something else.

Reader 2:   Then the Lord said to me, "Don't I have the right to do with you people of Israel what the potter did with the clay? You are in my hands just like clay in the potter's hands. If at any time I say that I am going to uproot, break down, or destroy any nation or kingdom, but then the nation turns from its evil, I will not do what I said I would. On the other hand, if I say that I am going to plant or build up any nation or kingdom, but then that nation disobeys me and does evil, I will not do what I said I would. . . . Don't I have the right to do with you people of Israel what the potter did with the clay?" (Jeremiah 18:1-10).

Reader 3: Just as clay is in the potter's hands for him to shape as he pleases, so we are in the hands of our Creator for him to do with as he wishes (Sirach 33:13).

The leader holds up clay, molded in a simple shape (cup, heart, wings, etc.) and explains that this shape represents what she or he wants God to shape in her or him.

Leader: **What is it that you want God to shape in *you*? Please take a moment to shape your own clay.**

The leader gives each participant a small piece of clay and plays instrumental music softly while the participants shape clay. The leader then asks each participant to explain what they have created.

Leader: **We are forever being formed. We never quite remain the same. Our joys and our sorrows mold us and shape us.**

The suffering we have gone through will keep our clay soft and yielding so that the Master Potter can continually and lovingly shape and re-shape us to his image—but only if we choose to remain moist and supple in his hands.

And so we ask for the capacity to use our sufferings in such a way that we are forever vulnerable to the shape that God has in mind for us.

All: May the God of strength be with us,
and keep us in strong-fingered hands:
may we be the sacrament of strength
to those whom we meet.
May the God of wonder be with us,
delighting us with thunder and wind, sunrise and rain,
enchanting our senses, filling our hearts,
and opening our eyes to the splendor of his creation.
May the God of patience be with us,
waiting for us with outstretched arms,
letting us find out for ourselves.
May the God of peace be with us,
stilling the heart that hammers
with fear, doubt, and confusion:
and may the warm mantle of his peace cover the anxious.

Final Blessing

Leader: **May the God of love be with us, drawing us close.**

All: May this love in us be for those we meet;
may this love glow in our eyes
and meet God's love reflected in the eyes of our friends
and especially those who, like us,
have suffered the loss of a loved one.

Leader: **May we always be open and pliant to what the Lord wants to mold in us. May we always be ready to allow the Divine Potter to gently shape us into a likeness of himself.**

All: Amen.

Let Our Clay Be Moist

Theme: Our suffering can allow the Lord to mold our lives into something new.

Introduction

Gathering Ritual

Reader 1: **The Lord said to me, "Go down to the potter's house, where I will give you my message." So I went there and saw the potter working at his wheel. Whenever a piece of pottery turned out imperfectly, he would take the clay and make it into something else.**

Reader 2: **Then the Lord said to me, "Don't I have the right to do with you people of Israel what the potter did with the clay? You are in my hands just like clay in the potter's hands. If at any time I say that I am going to uproot, break down, or destroy any nation or kingdom, but then the nation turns from its evil, I will not do what I said I would. On the other hand, if I say that I am going to plant or build up any nation or kingdom, but then that nation disobeys me and does evil, I will not do what I said I would. . . . Don't I have the right to do with you people of Israel what the potter did with the clay?"** (Jeremiah 18:1-10).

Reader 3: **Just as clay is in the potter's hands for him to shape as he pleases, so we are in the hands of our Creator for him to do with as he wishes** (Sirach 33:13).

Reflection

Leader: . . . we ask for the capacity to use our sufferings in such a way that we are forever vulnerable to the shape God has in mind for us.

All: **May the God of strength be with us,**
and keep us in strong-fingered hands:
may we be the sacrament of strength
to those whom we meet.
May the God of wonder be with us,
delighting us with thunder and wind, sunrise and rain,
enchanting our senses, filling our hearts,
and opening our eyes to the splendor of his creation.
May the God of patience be with us,
waiting for us with outstretched arms,
letting us find out for ourselves.
May the God of peace be with us,
stilling the heart that hammers
with fear, doubt, and confusion:
and may the warm mantle of his peace cover the anxious.

Final Blessing

Leader: May the God of love be with us, drawing us close.

All: **May this love in us be for those we meet;**
may this love glow in our eyes
and meet God's love reflected in the eyes of our friends
and especially those who, like us,
have suffered the loss of a loved one.

Leader: May we always be open and pliant to what the Lord wants to mold in us. May we always be ready to allow the Divine Potter to gently shape us into a likeness of himself.

All: **Amen.**

Heal Me, Lord

(For use at any time)

Theme: We need to ask the Lord to heal us of our suffering.

Materials Needed:

1. Music tape: "Be Not Afraid" *(Glory and Praise,* #8) (or simply read lyrics)—see "Resources Needed," p. 11.
2. Tape player
3. Some kind of oil in a bowl
4. Tissues to wipe oil after anointing

Introduction

Leader: **We are all aware of the healing and strengthening properties of oil. For centuries, athletes have rubbed their bodies with oil before beginning a race or taking part in a competition. Mothers rub oil on their babies to keep their bodies healthy. The church uses oil as a symbol of strength and healing in the sacraments of ordination, confirmation, and anointing of the sick.**

When we are bathed in oil, we feel comforted, rested, and eased of our pains.

Today we ask the Lord to comfort us and bless us as we struggle to move beyond our pain and face a life that will be new for us.

Let us read the words of Jeremiah the prophet as we pray for healing and strength.

All: Heal me, O Lord, and I shall be healed;
save me and I shall be saved;
for you are my praise . . .
you are my refuge in time of disaster.
(Jeremiah 17:14, 17b)

Gathering Ritual and Reflection

Leader: **Let us read together the words of Isaiah.**

All: The spirit of the Lord God is upon me,
because the Lord has anointed me;
He has sent me to bring good news to the oppressed,

to bind up the brokenhearted . . .
to provide for those who mourn in Zion . . .
to give them oil . . . of gladness instead of mourning,
the mantle of praise instead of a faint spirit.
(Isaiah 61:1, 3)

Leader: **Once again, we hear of the healing power of oil. The Lord God says he will give us the "oil of gladness in place of mourning."**

We come before the Lord with hearts filled with many emotions. We are happy to be in his presence, and to feel the understanding and compassion of all those who are gathered with us. And yet, we somehow know we are in need of an inner healing. We are searching for the ability to let go of our enormous suffering so that we can begin to grow through the sorrows we have experienced.

And so together, let us dip our fingers in the oil that is placed before us and ask the Lord to heal us and strengthen us as we anoint ourselves.

Each participant is invited to dip a finger in the oil and sign the various parts of the body as the leader reads.

Leader: **Anoint my head so that all my thoughts may be your thoughts, O Lord.**

Anoint my eyes so that I may see your Presence in what has happened in my life.

Anoint my ears that I may bear the cries of others who are suffering.

Anoint my lips that I may speak to those who struggle alongside me on this journey of grief.

Anoint my heart with compassion that I may be open to the sufferings of others.

The leader asks each participant to turn to the person beside him or her and anoint his or her forehead.

All: Anoint my companion with oil, O God,
that she/he may be healthy and strong
on (her/his) journey through grief.
In the name of the Father and of the Son and of the Holy Spirit. Amen.

Leader: **There are many people in our lives who need healing and strength. Let us pray together, naming those for whom we would like to pray.**

The leader allows a few moments for the participants to mention their intentions.

Leader concludes:

Lord, hear our prayers.

Final Blessing

Leader: **We have anointed each other with the oil of healing and strength. Let us listen for a moment to what the Lord promises each one of us, his anointed ones:**

The leader leads group in singing or reading the words of "Be Not Afraid."

Leader: **When you pass through the waters, I will be with you;**
and through the rivers, they shall not overwhelm you;
when you walk through fire you shall not be burned,
and the flame shall not consume you.
For I am the Lord your God,
the Holy One of Israel, your Savior.
(Isaiah 43:2-3)

Heal Me, Lord

Heal Me, Lord

Theme: We need to ask the Lord to heal us of our suffering.

Introduction

All: **Heal me, O Lord, and I shall be healed;**
save me and I shall be saved;
for you are my praise . . .
you are my refuge in time of disaster.
(Jeremiah 17:14, 17b)

Gathering Ritual and Reflection

Leader: Let us read together the words of Isaiah.

All: **The spirit of the Lord God is upon me,**
because the Lord has anointed me;
He has sent me to bring good news to the oppressed,
to bind up the brokenhearted . . .
to provide for those who mourn in Zion . . .
to give them oil . . . of gladness instead of mourning,
the mantle of praise instead of a faint spirit.
(Isaiah 61:1, 3)

All: **Anoint my companion with oil, O God,**
that (she/he) may be healthy and strong
on (her/his) journey through grief.
In the name of the Father and of the Son and of the Holy
Spirit. Amen.

Final Blessing

Voices of Grief, Voices of Healing

(This prayer service is especially appropriate for
participants who have spent some time in the grieving process
and are ready to face new life and new challenges.)

Materials Needed:

1. Music tape: "We Remember," Marty Haugen (see "Resources Needed," p. 11) or instrumental music
2. Tape player

In preparation for this service, the leader should seek out several participants who have recently experienced, and begun to recover from, a grief experience. Each of these should be asked to share very briefly about their experience of grief and then about their experience of healing. An explanatory page (with examples), following this service, may be duplicated and given to these participants.

Opening Prayer

Leader: **Loving God of life, death, and resurrection,**
we acknowledge your presence within us and among us.
As we gather before you, we remember and thank you
for the times you have been with us in our life.
As we recall our loved ones who have gone before us,
we ask you to give us ears to hear
the many voices of grief in this world
and the wisdom to respond with care and concern to them,
so that soon those voices may be strengthened and healed.
We ask this in Jesus' name. Amen.

The leader plays "We Remember" or instrumental music.

All: "We remember how you loved us to your death,
and still we celebrate, for you are with us here;
And we believe that we will see you
when you come in your glory, Lord,
we remember, we celebrate, we believe.

"Here, a million wounded souls
are yearning just to touch you and be healed;
Gather all your people, and hold them to your heart."[11]

Voices of Grief

Leader: **Christ said: "Blessed are they who mourn." Let us listen to the voices of those who have grieved their loved ones.**

Those who have agreed to share describe their experiences of grief.

Voices of Healing

Leader: **Christ concluded the beatitude "Blessed are they who mourn . . ." with the words ". . . for they shall be comforted."**

Let us listen to the voices of those who received comfort in the midst of their grieving and now look forward to new life.

Those who have agreed to share describe their experiences of healing.

All: "We remember how you loved us to your death,
and still we celebrate, for you are with us here;
And we believe that we will see you
when you come in your glory, Lord,
we remember, we celebrate, we believe.

"See the Face of Christ revealed in every person standing by your side;
Gift to one another, and temples of your love."[12]

Leader: **Let us pray.**

All: Heavenly Father, we have listened to the voices of grief
that we are so familiar with.
Some of those voices are our own.
But we are strengthened by the voices of healing
because we have begun to realize
that with the help and comfort of those around us,
those voices can be ours also.
Continue to be with us on our grief journey
so that we can find the peace and joy
that comes to those who seek you through their sorrow.
Amen.

PRAYING THROUGH GRIEF

Voices of Grief, Voices of Healing

Opening Prayer

All: "We remember how you loved us to your death,
and still we celebrate, for you are with us here;
And we believe that we will see you
when you come, in your glory, Lord,
we remember, we celebrate, we believe.

"Here, a million wounded souls
are yearning just to touch you and be healed;
Gather all your people, and hold them to your heart."*

Voices of Grief

Voices of Healing

All: "We remember how you loved us to your death,
and still we celebrate, for you are with us here;
And we believe that we will see you
when you come, in your glory, Lord,
we remember, we celebrate, we believe.

"See the Face of Christ revealed in every person
standing by your side;
Gift to one another, and temples of your love."*

Leader: Let us pray.

All: Heavenly Father, we have listened to the voices of grief
that we are so familiar with.
Some of those voices are our own.
But we are strengthened by the voices of healing
because we have begun to realize
that with the help and comfort of those around us,

those voices can be ours also.
Continue to be with us on our grief journey
so that we can find the peace and joy
that comes to those who seek you through their sorrow.
Amen.

* "We Remember," Marty Haugen. G.I.A. publications, Inc., 7404 S. Mason Ave., Chicago, IL 60638. Permission granted for duplication.

"Voices of Grief, Voices of Healing" Prayer Service

Explanation to Volunteers

Thank you for agreeing to share your experiences of loss and of healing in our service of prayer. You will be asked to share very briefly at two different times in the service.

First, you will be asked to give a short description of the grief you experienced. Here are some examples that may help you to formulate your thoughts:

(Woman who lost husband)

> "John and I were married almost fifty-two years when he had a heart attack and died. I remember that people told me I was lucky because I had him so long. But, the longer I had him the more I loved him . . . and the harder I grieved because he's no longer with me."

(Father who lost son)

> "For fifteen years I was always there for Bobby, especially if he got hurt or was in trouble. I was always able to fix things up for him. But when he was hit by the car on that icy afternoon, I remember that I wasn't there—and I couldn't fix him because he was already dead when I got to the hospital."

(Girl who lost sister)

> "I remember how my sister and I used to fight over whose turn it was to do the dishes. And then my sister died of cancer, and now I feel mean because I fought with her and I wish it never happened."

(Man who lost co-worker)

> "I remember how Brad and I used to eat lunch together and argue about politics, football teams, and most other things in life. And now he is dead and somehow lunch doesn't mean anything to me any more; I'd just as soon skip it."

(Young man who lost friend to suicide)

> "I don't understand Chris. I remember when we talked about how we'd go to college together and be roommates. And now he's gone, and I don't even want to think about having somebody else as a roommate."

(Person with cancer)

> "I remember how I used to be able to do everything at all hours of the day and night. People always thought I was younger than I was. And now my body is getting older very quickly as cancer takes its toll. I'm scared."

Second, you will be asked to describe some experience of healing or comfort. Here are some examples:

(Woman who lost husband)

> "I remember what my pharmacist said to me when I told him I wouldn't be renewing John's prescription because he had died. He said: `Mary, John was such a kind man. What a great pair you made.' And I was happy to know someone considered us a great pair. I did!"

(Father who lost son)

> "I remember reading in a book someone recommended to me when my son died, something that really helped me: `We are offered the choice between two gift-wrapped packages with grief: one filled with bitterness and anger, one filled with blessings. Both gifts change your life.' I guess I am the one who needs to make the right choice."

(Girl who lost sister)

> "My teacher was really cool when my sister died. She didn't say anything when I went back to school after the funeral. She just put her arms around me, and even cried with me. She really cared about me without ever having to tell me that."

(Man who lost co-worker)

> "I went to a support group after Brad died. I just couldn't handle my best friend who was exactly my age not being around any more. The group was great. Most of them had lost their wives or their husbands, but they treated me who had lost just a friend, as if my grief was as great as theirs. They seemed to realize losing anyone you cared about was a terrible thing."

(Young man who lost friend to suicide)

> "A lot of us were very upset when we learned Chris had committed suicide. One of the priests from Chris's parish came to the wake, and afterward, he got all of Chris's friends together, and we went out for pizza. We all talked about Chris and the great times we had together. It was so good to hear some of the stories the other kids told. And I got to tell some too—and I really feel better now, even though I don't understand why Chris had to take his own life."

(Person with cancer)

"It's been so hard for me to talk to my family about my cancer. They don't want to even think about my death, which I know will be soon. But the visiting nurse who comes to give me shots three times a week has been wonderful to me. She lets me talk and listens to me very carefully. It's so great to have someone listen to me when I am so scared."

Endnotes

1. Adapted from "The Sycamore Retreat," *Mortal on the Mend,* Vincent Marquis, Wallingford, CT (unpublished).

2. Adapted from *Gift from the Sea,* Anne Morrow Lindbergh (Pantheon Books, 1955), pp. 21-22.

3. Adapted from *Praying Our Goodbyes,* Joyce Rupp (Ave Maria Press, 1988), p. 176.

4. "We Remember," Marty Haugen (G.I.A. Publications).

5. "We Remember," Marty Haugen (G.I.A. Publications).

6. *Gift from the Sea,* Anne Morrow Lindbergh (Pantheon Books, 1955), p. 116.

7. "Light a Candle," Paul Alexander (Paul Alexander Music, 1993).

8. *Mortal on the Mend,* Vincent Marquis, Wallingford, CT (unpublished).

9. *Mortal on the Mend,* Vincent Marquis, Wallingford, CT (unpublished).

10. Excerpted from *Gates of Prayer* (Reformed Jewish Prayerbook), p. 552.

11. "We Remember," Marty Haugen (G.I.A. Publications).

12. "We Remember," Marty Haugen (G.I.A. Publications).